Whittle
BOOKS

WHITTLE BOOKS IN ASSOCIATION WITH
PENGUIN BOOKS

THE LOGIC OF HEALTH CARE REFORM

Paul Starr served as an adviser to the White House during the development of the Clinton health plan and has
been described by *The New York Times* and other pub-
lications as one of the plan's architects. He is coeditor of
The American Prospect, a liberal journal of public policy and social criticism, and author of *The Social
Transformation of American Medicine*, which received
the Pulitzer Prize for general nonfiction, the Bancroft
Prize in American history, the James Hamilton Award of
the American College of Health Care Executives, and
the C. Wright Mills Award of the Society for the Study
of Social Problems. The first edition of *The Logic of
Health Care Reform*, originally subtitled *Transforming
American Medicine for the Better*, was published by
Grand Rounds Press in October 1992. Starr has written
on politics, public policy, and American society for mag-
azines and academic journals. He and his wife, Sandra,
have four children.

THE LOGIC OF HEALTH CARE REFORM

WHY AND HOW THE PRESIDENT'S PLAN WILL WORK

REVISED AND EXPANDED EDITION

Paul Starr

WHITTLE BOOKS
IN ASSOCIATION WITH
PENGUIN BOOKS

PENGUIN BOOKS
Published by the Penguin Group Penguin Books USA Inc., 375 Hudson Street,
New York, New York 10014, U.S.A.
Penguin Books Ltd, 27 Wrights Lane, London W8 5TZ, England
Penguin Books Australia Ltd, Ringwood, Victoria, Australia
Penguin Books Canada Ltd, 10 Alcorn Avenue,
Toronto, Ontario, Canada M4V 3B2
Penguin Books (N.Z.) Ltd, 182-190 Wairau Road, Auckland 10, New Zealand

Penguin Books Ltd, Registered Offices:
Harmondsworth, Middlesex, England

This revised and updated edition first published in Penguin Books 1994

1 3 5 7 9 10 8 6 4 2

This book was first published by Whittle Books as part of The Grand Rounds
Press series. Published by arrangement with
Whittle Communications L.P.

Charts: Linda Eckstein. Sources: *Health Affairs*, Summer 1990 and Fall 1991 (data
from Harvard-Harris-ITF 1990 Ten-Nation Survey and OECD Health Data, 1991),
page 4; "EBRI Special Report and Issue Brief Number 145," January 1994 (data
from Current Population Survey, March 1993), page 7; Alliance for Health Reform, "Health Care in America," May 1992 (based on "ERBI Issue Brief," February 1991), page 11; HCFA, National Center for Education Statistics and *Statistical
Abstract of the United States*, 19th edition, page 13; *Health Affairs*, Fall 1991 and
Summer 1993 (based on *OECD Health Systems: Facts and Trends*, 1993), page
18; *Medical Economics*, November 4, 1991, page 20; AMA's *Physician Characteristics in the U.S., 1992*, page 33; U.S. Congressional Budget Office (based on
data from *Health Affairs*, Winter 1991), page 38; Paul Starr, page 51; U.S. General Accounting Office report, "Private Health Insurance: Problems Caused by a
Segmented Market," July 1991, page 58; KPMG Peat Marwick, page 68; Clinton
administration, pages 72 and 75; Paul Starr, page 74.

Library of Congress Catalog Card Number: 92-85362
ISBN 0 14 02.3893 X

Printed in the United States of America
Set in Sabon
Based on a design by Kathryn Parise

To Rebecca, Olivia, Raphael, and Abigail

ACKNOWLEDGMENTS

Writing requires cooperation, tolerance, and forgiveness, especially if the writer has a large family and diligent editors. I am indebted not only to them but to a number of people who took the time (when there wasn't much) to give me comments on the original manuscript even though they may have disagreed in significant respects. I would like to thank Linda Bergthold, Alain Enthoven, Alan Hillman, Jon Kingsdale, Theodore R. Marmor, Jeremy Rosner, Steven Schroeder, Shoshanna Sofaer, Harold Stein, and Walter Zelman. I regret that I could not take all their suggestions, although I reserve that right for future projects. This book also reflects the many ideas of my wife, Sandra, who helped think about the book before a word was written.

CONTENTS

Contents

INTRODUCTION

TO THE PENGUIN EDITION

This has become a different book since its original publication in October 1992. The ideas are the same, but they are no longer as much my own. Nor do they belong any more to the loose network of reformers who developed similar proposals in the months leading up to the 1992 election and after. In the space of a year, the approach presented in these pages has traveled from the margins to the center of national debate. The ideas have been turned from a conceptual framework into a detailed plan, and then from a plan into legislation, presented to Congress by President Clinton.

Along the way, there have been plenty of changes in specific features of the plan, and more will undoubtedly come. This book is for people who want to understand the basic paradigm of reform proposed by the President and come to a judgment about how it will work.

Some may also be curious about how the approach adopted by the President came to influence national policy. Fragments of the story have appeared in the news media, inevitably dramatizing conflicts among personalities in the inner circles of power; book-length, behind-the-scenes accounts by journalists are on their way. Without claiming to tell the whole story, I can shed some light on the evolution of the ideas behind the policies.

The Turn Toward a New Paradigm

As a historically minded sociologist, I am inclined to emphasize patterns of long-term development that shape major changes in social institutions on the scale of national health reform. Deeply rooted economic and political forces are driving the reform of health insurance and health care in America. But as a participant in the process, I know (at least I think I know) that the election of Bill Clinton is the immediate reason for the emergence of a plan for universal health insurance based on "competition under a cap."

In early 1992, the news media generally presented a menu for reform of health care that had three major alternatives: a Canadian-style, single-payer system of national health insurance; the conservative approach proposed by President Bush to give tax credits for limited coverage to the poor in a modestly reformed insurance market; and play-or-pay, the proposal embraced by many large corporations and congressional Democrats, which requires employers to cover their workers or pay into a public insurance program. If a fourth possibility, managed competition, was ever mentioned, it was confused with conservative, free-market ideas (even "pure" managed competition has a lot more regulation than its advocates now generally admit). A universal health insurance plan that combined competition and a budget cap on health spending was not on the menu at all.

Getting airtime for a new approach wasn't easy. On May 6, 1992, I testified before the Senate Finance Committee, along with three economists: Karen Davis, a supporter of a single-payer approach and health care price regulation; Mark Pauly, who was close to the Bush administration; and Alain Enthoven, managed competition's chief architect. In my testimony (later incorporated into this book), I argued for universal coverage with private plans competing under a budget, and I highlighted a proposal for a publicly financed system of competing health plans introduced the previous February by John

Garamendi, California's elected Insurance Commissioner.[1] Looking back today, a reader of those hearings would realize I was describing the framework of what has since become the Clinton Health Security plan. But at the time it was just one of many ideas for reform. Major groups were not sponsoring it, national politicians were not supporting it, and the media were not spotlighting it.

Interest in this alternative model began to grow that spring and summer. A week after the Senate Finance hearing, Pennsylvania Senator Harris Wofford invited me to his office to meet Garamendi and his deputy, Walter Zelman, for a discussion about the Garamendi plan and an approach to national reform that gave the states a variety of options for carrying out universal coverage. (Garamendi had worked under Wofford three decades earlier, when Wofford was running the Peace Corps mission in Ethiopia.) We were joined by Senators Tom Daschle of South Dakota and Bob Kerrey of Nebraska and then met with a group of Washington health care reporters to discuss the Garamendi plan. Along with New Mexico Senator Jeff Bingaman, who had introduced a managed competition plan of his own, these were the members of the Senate who initially showed the most interest in an approach to universal coverage that provided for private plans competing under a budget and left a lot of flexibility to the states.

Among private organizations, the Catholic Health Association had developed a proposal that was the clos-

1. Testimony before the Committee on Finance, U.S. Senate, in *Comprehensive Health Care Reform and Cost Containment*, Hearings, 102d Cong., 2d sess., May 6, 1992, pp. 36–38, 389–393. For the Garamendi plan, see John Garamendi, "California Health Care in the 21st Century: A Vision for Reform," Department of Insurance, State of California, Febrary 1992. The plan has been stymied by California Governor Pete Wilson and the state's deep recession.

est to the new model.[2] It too called for competing plans under a budget, but like the proposal that Senator Kerrey had introduced in 1991, it envisioned paying health plans a fixed amount, allowing them to compete on quality but not on price.

Meanwhile, on a separate track, Enthoven, the physician Paul Ellwood, and Lynn Etheredge, a health policy consultant, were spearheading an effort based in Jackson Hole, Wyoming, to garner support for their model of "pure" managed competition, which rejected any expenditure caps or price controls.[3] During 1992 the Jackson Hole proposals drew editorial backing from *The New York Times* and favorable attention in *Business Week, Fortune,* and elsewhere. In the House of Representatives, conservative Democrats led by Jim Cooper of Tennessee were developing a managed competition bill incorporating Jackson Hole ideas but with one crucial omission: Cooper's bill omitted a mandate on employers to pay for health insurance and consequently did not provide for universal coverage. I had no involvement with these efforts and only read the Jackson Hole papers and Cooper bill, which was introduced in September, after I had finished a first draft of this book. The distinctive contribution of the Jackson Hole Group, it then seemed to me, was its emphasis on holding health plans accountable for quality as well as cost (hence the term "accountable health plan"); however, the group's approach did not strike me as recognizing the limits of a competitive market in either controlling costs or providing access for all Americans.

2. Catholic Health Association of the United States, "Setting Relationships Right: A Working Proposal for Systemic Healthcare Reform," February 20, 1992.

3. Jackson Hole Group, "The 21st Century American Health System," Policy Documents 1–4, 1991–1992.

My interest in an approach to national health insurance that relies on competition among prepaid health plans and countervailing purchasing power to control costs dates back to the 1970s.[4] As I worked on *The Social Transformation of American Medicine*—a historical account of the formation of the medical profession and related institutions—one of my concerns was to explain the forces that had shaped the health care and insurance industries in the late nineteenth and twentieth centuries, inhibiting the development of prepaid health plans, weakening the power of the purchasers, and blocking *both* effective competition and national health insurance.[5]

After that book's publication, I moved away from specific work on health care and became more generally concerned with the relation between the public and private sectors and the revival and reframing of liberal thought. In 1989, together with the columnist Robert Kuttner and Robert B. Reich, now Secretary of Labor, I founded *The American Prospect*, a magazine devoted to recasting liberal ideas about politics and public policy. As coeditor of *The American Prospect* I came to work with some of the people who have since become prominent in the Clinton administration and became concerned about linking good policy to successful politics.[6]

4. See Paul Starr, "The Undelivered Health System," *The Public Interest* No. 42 (Winter 1976), pp. 66–85, and "Controlling Medical Costs Through Countervailing Power," *Working Papers for a New Society* 5 (Summer 1977), pp. 10–11, 97–98.

5. See especially Book One, Chapter 6, and Book Two, Chapters 1–4, in *The Social Transformation of American Medicine* (New York: Basic Books, 1982).

6. In addition to Reich, *The American Prospect*'s writers have included Laura Tyson, chair of the Council of Economic Advisers; Alan Blinder, a member of the Council; Stanley B. Greenberg, the President's pollster; Alicia Munnell, assistant secretary of the Treasury; and Steven Kelman,

Then in 1991, as the rise in health costs and unravelling of the insurance system enlarged the constituency for health care reform, I came full-circle back to the ideas for reform I had written about fifteen years earlier.

When I distributed copies of the manuscript of *The Logic of Health Care Reform*, Reich was one of the readers. At the time, he and Ira Magaziner were playing central roles in shaping Clinton's economic program. Magaziner, a prominent business consultant, knew Reich and Clinton from their days as Rhodes scholars; he and Reich were coauthors of the 1982 book *Minding America's Business*, and they collaborated on the Clinton campaign book, *Putting People First*. Reich suggested I talk to Magaziner, who had recently been asked by Governor Clinton to do an independent review of health care reform for the presidential campaign. (Magaziner had just finished a study of health care and related services for the aged in his native Rhode Island.) In a phone conversation on July 18, Magaziner questioned me about the approach I was taking. The following Monday I sent him a copy of my manuscript, along with other materials he had asked to see. We continued to talk on and off over the next several weeks about the development of Clinton's position on health reform in the campaign's final months.

In candidate forums and position papers during the primaries, Clinton had already made clear his approach

director of procurement at the Office of Management and Budget. The policy-politics connection is evident in a series of articles about designing policies to meet the concerns of people who "work, pay taxes, and play by the rules" and thereby bring what Greenberg calls the "working middle class" back to the Democratic party. See Greenberg's "From Crisis to Working Majority," *The American Prospect* (Fall 1991), pp. 104–117, and my own "The Middle Class and National Health Reform," *The American Prospect* (Summer 1991), pp. 7–12.

without endorsing a specific bill in Congress. Rereading his campaign white paper on health care issued during the New Hampshire primary, I am struck by how closely the Clinton Health Security plan presented to Congress in the fall of 1993 tracks the specific points that Clinton raised as a candidate.[7]

The white paper called for universal coverage with a guaranteed benefits package, employment-based financing, cost containment in part through global budgeting, the use of health networks as an option for providing services, an emphasis on preventive and primary care, and an expansion of long-term care emphasizing care in the home. The paper does refer, however, to setting reimbursement rates for all payers and suggests that employers would have a play-or-pay choice either to cover their workers or to pay into a public program. These provisions are inconsistent with an approach that emphasizes managed competition and do not appear in the Clinton Health Security plan introduced in 1993.

A play-or-pay system poses financial risks that no government should accept. If employers have a choice about entering a public program, the employers that stay out will be those with relatively low health costs, and the public program will have a higher-risk, higher-cost enrollment. In addition, under the usual play-or-pay proposals, employers entering the public program would pay a payroll tax (estimates were running from 7 to 9 percent), while the employers outside could self-insure or pay premiums. As a result, the public program would tend to attract employers not only with above-average risks but also with below-average wages. Endemically underfinanced, the government program would almost certainly become a fiscal albatross and a

7. "Bill Clinton's American Health Care Plan," Little Rock, Ark., n.d.

source of inferior coverage. Furthermore, consumers would have no choice about whether to enroll; their employers would decide.

These objections weighed heavily with Magaziner. Still, to reject play-or-pay conspicuously in the midst of the campaign was impossible. The press would have called it a flipflop, and too many leading Democrats were committed to the approach. That summer it was unclear whether Clinton needed to pursue health policy in any greater detail; he had already said a lot. Polls indicated that the public overwhelmingly preferred him to Bush on health care. This was not a matter of support for a specific policy; the public generally trusted Democrats more than Republicans on the issue. Why become enmeshed in the details when what counted was the commitment? Besides, some argued, health care finance poses extremely complicated problems, and the heat of a campaign is not the best environment for resolving them. This was a legitimate and sensible position.

On the other hand, the press and various experts were berating Clinton for not fully specifying his plans to reform health care, and the Republicans were warming up for an attack on play-or-pay as threatening a 9 percent payroll tax and a back door to a government-run health system.

To broaden the range of views being heard in the campaign, Magaziner convened a meeting in Washington on Monday, August 10. For the first time, the campaign's Washington-based health policy advisory committee, notably including Judith Feder and Kenneth Thorpe, met with a number of people from around the country sympathetic to a managed competition approach, such as Zelman and Lois Quam, who had directed a reform effort in Minnesota. The session was chaired by Atul

Gawande, the young aide in charge of health issues in Little Rock.

The Clinton campaign was the natural place for health policy crossfertilization to take place. Clinton sought to unite more traditional liberals with "new Democrats." As director of the bipartisan Pepper Commission, an effort that sought unsuccessfully to build consensus for health care reform, Judith Feder had worked for Senator Jay Rockefeller; Atul Gawande had previously worked for Representative Cooper. A reform plan that combined the security of universal, comprehensive coverage with consumer choice and competition in the delivery of services was, in a sense, the natural byproduct of the Democratic party that Bill Clinton was trying to put back together. All along, it has been a question of the balance between the two sides of the party and the policy (and whether they could stick together!).

The discussion at the Washington meeting was intense, but Feder and others in the advisory group did not reject a competitive approach as long as it had a regulatory backup.[8] Under Magaziner's gentle prodding, a fragile consensus in favor of a half turn toward managed competition emerged from the Washington meeting, and the next month, a small delegation from the campaign discussed the new option with Clinton on the campaign trail in East Lansing, Michigan. Soon after, on September 24, in a speech in New Jersey and an accompanying press release from Little Rock, Clinton called for universal health coverage "privately provided, publicly guaranteed" under a system of "competition within a budget." The news media did not understand that he

8. Thorpe was also developing a combined approach to cost containment: Kenneth E. Thorpe, "The Best of Both Worlds: Merging Competition and Regulation," *Journal of American Health Policy* (July/August 1992), pp. 20–24.

was signaling an important step. "Competition within a budget" didn't register; it was not one of the familiar choices on their menu. After a skeptical *New York Times* editorial and some grief in Little Rock, the campaign issued "talking points" to clarify that Clinton did not envision price controls, and the *Times* declared victory for managed competition. During the first debate with President Bush and Ross Perot, Clinton responded to a question about health care by immediately referring to his "managed competition" plan. I wondered how many people across America had any idea what he meant.

It seems improbable that Clinton's embrace of competition had any effect on the election. Bush muffed questions about health care reform during the debates, and his campaign never aired television spots that it had prepared on health care, apparently concluding that they would only highlight an issue on which Bush did not enjoy public trust. Yet Clinton's September turn toward competition within a budget did matter a great deal after the election. It guided the work that led to the Health Security plan, presented to Congress almost exactly one year later, on September 23, 1993.

From Paradigm to Plan (1): Getting Started

The distance between a conceptual paradigm and a detailed plan to carry it out is enormous, and many a concept has not survived the trip. If "competition under a cap" was to become a serious contender for national policy, it needed a lot more work than anyone had yet done.

Just before and after the '92 election, I tried to advance that work through a project that had grown out of the meeting with Garamendi and Zelman in May: a conference on universal health insurance and managed competition at Princeton in late November, funded by the Robert Wood Johnson Foundation before Clinton became associated with the approach. My aim was to follow up the first edition of this book by assembling a group of policy experts who could begin answering in detail many of the hard questions that had to be confronted: What benefits would be covered? How would the new system be financed? How would the new health insurance purchasing cooperatives be organized and governed? What would be the relation between the federal government and the states? I worked closely with Zelman and several people who had advised him on the Garamendi plan, including Larry Levitt, Rick Kronick, and Linda Bergthold.

It was out of a meeting with this group in California on October 27 that a key idea emerged for financing coverage. The Garamendi plan relied primarily on a payroll tax; I had taken the same approach in the first edition of this book, while mentioning in just one paragraph that the system could also be financed by premiums. In September, Clinton had publicly ruled out a payroll tax. The alternative we discussed in California was a "capped" premium. Employers and individuals would each owe a share of the premium, with employer contributions capped as a percentage of payroll and individual contributions capped as a percentage of family income. Like play-or-pay, this approach would limit employers' liabilities to either a percentage of a premium or a flat proportion of payroll (whichever was lower), but it avoided creating a separate public program with a high-cost, low-wage population. After the California meeting, I arranged with the consulting firm Lewin-VHI to cost out the capped premium approach, according to my own primitive specifications. The Lewin numbers were, I believe, the first estimates—at least the first to be made public—of the kind of approach to financing coverage eventually taken by the Clinton Health Security plan.[9]

Clinton's election victory and the growing recognition of his interest in the approach lent the late November conference in Princeton an air of high expectation. Many of the key congressional staff members concerned with health legislation took part; ten other participants, including six authors of papers, went on to work on the White House effort a few months later. Not all the participants who favored a competitive system, such as Enthoven, approved of budget caps; not all who favored budget caps, such as Henry Aaron, had any faith in competition. While prefiguring difficult debates to come, the discussion and the fourteen papers presented—all but two of them published in a supplement of the journal *Health Affairs* four and a half months later—began to give the model sharper definition and more credibility.[10]

The project fulfilled its purpose in a way I had not expected. Like other transition groups, the presidential transition group on health policy, led by Judith Feder, did not issue a public report. In the first half year of the new administration, the same was true for the presidential task force and working groups set up to study alternatives. As a result, there was little available for anyone to read about the approach to health care reform of the new administration. Along with *The Logic of Health*

9. John F. Sheils, Lawrence S. Lewin, and Randall A. Haught, "Potential Public Expenditures under Managed Competition," *Health Affairs* (Supplement 1993), pp. 229–242. Enthoven was the host for the California meeting, but he was not a proponent of this approach.

10. An overview, "A Bridge to Compromise: Competition Within a Budget," *Health Affairs* (Supplement 1993), pp. 7–23, which I wrote with Zelman, sums up where we stood just before the work of the new administration began.

Care Reform and a subsequent *American Prospect* article,[11] the papers from the Princeton conference helped to fill that vacuum, though they never had any official benediction.

Still, the Princeton papers were at a high level of generality; they left innumerable political and technical questions unresolved. They also focused on a more narrow set of issues than Clinton had addressed in his campaign. The circle of people involved was extremely limited. And the language being used was intelligible only to health policy experts. The next steps would have to move in several directions simultaneously. The new administration would have to broaden the range of issues and people involved; it would need both more complex analytical work on the policy and simpler ways to explain it. At the time, I did not understand all that needed doing. Fortunately, President Clinton turned to people who did.

From Paradigm to Plan (2): The Presidential Phase

In early January, the President-elect asked Magaziner to organize a comprehensive reform initiative in the White House that would be chaired and led by Mrs. Clinton. Announced a few days after the inauguration, the effort took the form of a small task force composed primarily of members of the Cabinet and a supporting cast that ultimately included hundreds of people organized into more than thirty "working groups." In the last week of January, while I was in Washington to speak to a congressional breakfast meeting and a conference run by the grass-roots organization Citizen Action, Magaziner asked me to come on board as one of the working group

11. "Healthy Compromise: Universal Coverage and Managed Competition Under a Cap," *The American Prospect*, No. 12, Winter 1993, pp. 44–52.

leaders. It was "showtime" for health care reform, he said. I was there the next day for the first organizational meeting with Mrs. Clinton.

With the task force originally due to report in 100 days, the working groups and White House staff concerned with health care started off at a feverish pace, operating from daybreak until near midnight in what seemed like nonstop meetings. The group leaders had been recruited from the earlier campaign advisory committee and presidential transition team, from the network of people who had worked on the Garamendi plan and the Princeton conference, and from the various Cabinet departments concerned with health care: principally the Departments of Health and Human Services (HHS), Labor, Treasury, Veterans Affairs (VA), and Defense as well as the Office of Management and Budget (OMB) and the Council of Economic Advisers. My initial responsibility was to supervise one of the "clusters" comprising three working groups: short-term cost controls, administrative simplification, and phase-in of the new system. I also worked closely with the cluster concerned with the new system's structure.

The participants in the working groups were generally chosen for their technical knowledge, not because they were true believers. Most were regular employees of federal agencies; a small minority were "temps," as I was. (I had taken a one-semester leave and would return to Princeton in the fall.) Among the members were people representing a diversity of backgrounds and professions, including some sixty physicians. Also invited to join the groups were dozens of congressional staff (Democrats only), as well as a smaller number of people sent by governors (both Democrats and Republicans) via the National Governors Association. This breadth of participation was extraordinary. Policymaking efforts of the executive branch do not normally include legislative staff, much less representatives of the states.

Yet in one respect, this outreach had the opposite effect from what was intended. Private interest groups protested their exclusion—there were individual doctors but no representatives of the American Medical Association—and the press was outraged that the groups at the White House met behind "closed doors." Of course, no one had seemed to mind when previous presidents developed policies behind closed doors at the White House. What president had ever done otherwise? The irony was that the very effort to include so many people had produced a deeper sense of exclusion among those who were left out, especially the press.

Furthermore, not much was kept secret. Any paper distributed at working group meetings quickly found its way to the news media. Memos that had no standing whatsoever as administration policy generated newspaper stories that began "The Clinton administration is considering . . ." The result was hyperbolic confusion over what the administration was going to propose.

Much of the media coverage reflected a misunderstanding of the process. During the winter and most of the spring, there was a deliberate separation of policy and politics. The members of the working groups writing memos on the pros and cons of alternative policies simply did not know which might be seriously considered. They had only the broadest political guidance, based on what the President had said in the campaign. Meanwhile, others at the White House, generally veterans of the 1992 campaign, were concerned with communications, interest group liaison, relations with Congress and the governors, and overall political strategy. Magaziner and a few others spanned the two sides of the process; eventually the pieces would come together. In fact, no final decisions could take place until the technical work on policy was joined with a broader political understanding. (A good plan for reform that could not be passed was not a good plan.) It was not the job of the working groups to make those defining judgments, nor should it have been, yet many of the people involved were frustrated by the inherently ambiguous direction they received.

At the outset, many aspects of the ultimate form of the administration's plan were uncertain. Subsequent reports in the media have suggested that the plan had already been decided on and that the entire effort was only a charade; other articles have portrayed a White House bouncing from one option to another. Neither of these views captures what really happened. There were diverse voices within the administration; the working groups included people whose views spanned the spectrum from a single-payer approach to "pure" managed competition. However, the President's statements during the campaign had effectively ruled out a tax-financed single-payer plan and pure competition.[12] From the beginning, the working group effort had a direction that was implicit in the focus on both competition and budget caps, but a wide range of alternatives remained open. The approach taken in the campaign did not, for example, rule out some short-term use of price controls until a competitive system could be organized. It did not

12. Soon after the establishment of the working groups, in an article spread across the front of its Sunday financial section, *The New York Times* described the Jackson Hole Group as Hillary Rodham Clinton's "brain trust." This claim had no factual basis. Among the leaders of the working group effort, there was only one member of the Jackson Hole Group (Thomas Pyle), and he soon left. Other articles in the *Times* have suggested that Enthoven was the "abandoned father" of reform, the "originator" of the idea later spurned. In fact, from the campaign onward, Clinton always spoke of competition

rule out allowing states the flexibility to carry out a national program through a single-payer system or all-payer rate setting. It did not resolve what to do about long-term care, mental health benefits, and many other questions. The process was open enough to allow fundamentally different alternatives to be floated and discussed—such as a value-added tax for financing—if only in the end to be shot down.

Magaziner had designed the working group effort on a model taken from his experience as a business consultant. The paradigm was a corporate restructuring or technological innovation that required thinking through innumerable options and suboptions and meshing together previously uncoordinated activities and groups into a coherent plan. The enormity of the project was evident in the organization of the working groups. Cluster 1 included groups concerned with the design of health insurance purchasing cooperatives, relations among health plans and providers, insurance market reform, budget caps, and special concerns of rural and inner-city areas. A second cluster dealt with coverage, benefits, low-income households, and Medicaid. Cluster 3 dealt with quality improvement, information systems, the health care workforce, and malpractice; a fourth cluster with the integration of current government programs: Medicare, the veterans' and military health care systems, and federal employees' health benefits. Other

---

"within a budget" He never embraced the Jackson Hole approach. During the campaign and development of the plan, we tried to convince the Jackson Hole Group to accept budget caps: Vast stretches of the country are unlikely to have any competition, and many areas will have no more than oligopolistic competition among a small number of plans. However, Enthoven and the others refuse to recognize these limits to their theory, and it should be no surprise that since the release of the Clinton plan they have opposed it.

clusters dealt with underserved and vulnerable populations, long-term care, and financing, and still other
groups performed general analytical functions: quantitative analysis, ethical evaluation, assessment of economic impacts, and legislative drafting.

The scale of the project was astonishing even to some
of us who had long advocated a comprehensive plan, and
rather than being scaled back, it expanded. The initial
design did not include separate groups on mental health
services, the Indian Health Service, or academic health
centers, and these were added. As the process unfolded,
external review groups were convened, consisting of
physicians, nurses, health care managers, actuaries, and
others, as well as panels of consumers who had written
letters to Mrs. Clinton.

According to Magaziner's design, the working groups
were initially to go through a "broadening" process to
ensure that all relevant issues and options were considered; then a "narrowing" phase to reduce the alternatives to a manageable set for decision making; and,
finally, auditing and criticism by contrarians and other
independent reviewers. To ensure progress along this
route, there was a schedule of "tollgates"—checkpoints
when periodic reports were due and the groups would
report back on the status of their work.

The tollgates will long be engraved in the memory of
the hundreds who took part in them. They generally
took place in the ornate Indian Treaty Room at the top
of the Old Executive Office Building overlooking the
White House and stretched on for entire days, even
through one weekend. The members of each cluster, the
largest of which included well over a hundred people,
would file into the room, and Magaziner and several
others of us who worked for him sat on folding chairs at
tables arranged in a large rectangle to hear the presenta-

tions and ask questions. The tollgates were marathon seminars, often technical and inconclusive, but the grandeur of the setting and the size of the meetings gave them a theatrical quality.

In February and March, the tollgates produced a great deal of high-quality analysis, pushing farther ahead than either the presidential transition or Princeton conference. Both larger principles and smaller details gradually came into focus as the groups worked methodically through the issues. As winter turned to spring, however, events beyond anyone's control created a stop-and-go pattern. Lawsuits over Mrs. Clinton's role in the task force (which was ultimately upheld by the courts) complicated the process. In March, the plan began to take shape through meetings with the President, Mrs. Clinton, and members of the Cabinet. Then the illness and death of Mrs. Clinton's father slowed progress. Later, task force meetings on the health plan stopped entirely because distorted leaks and rumors about financing threatened to disrupt passage of the President's budget in Congress.

At the end of May, the legal existence of the task force came to an end; by that time, the members of the working groups had dispersed. Magaziner continued to be in charge of developing the plan and was supported by the White House political strategy and communications team; a small policy group with offices at the White House; a cross-cutting "quantitative analysis" and budget group drawn from HHS, Treasury, the Council of Economic Advisers, and OMB; and the drafting group responsible for writing the legislation. A number of people overlapped or floated among more than one of these groups at various times, and the focal point of de facto policy making shifted. For example, during much of the spring, the quantitative analysis group was central, as alternative policies were analyzed for their effects on health premiums, government budgets, and the private sector.

Although there was an earlier version that never leaked, it was only at the end of May that the policy group began to write the reform plan in detail. The *Wall Street Journal* reported that I was responsible for writing the plan. This was not the case. (The confusion about my role arose because I had spent much of April and May writing an early draft of what was later issued, in a very different form, as *Health Security: The President's Report to the American People*.) Astonishingly, the policy group was able to work through the summer on the plan, known internally as the "policy book," without premature disclosures. Final decisions made at meetings at the end of August and beginning of September were incorporated in revisions written the following weekend. It was only when the policy book was sent to the Congress for consultations the next week that it finally leaked. Although never intended for public release (it includes little explanation of any policy), this preliminary draft of the plan is the version that first appeared in print and continues, as I write, to be the one most widely distributed.

How and why President Clinton made key decisions about the plan is a story that will have to wait. A time will come for a full history when there is a full history to be told. I can say this: The strength of conviction about health care reform that the American people heard in the President's voice when he spoke to the Congress the evening of September 23, 1993, I had heard before in meetings at the White House. I do not believe there was any historical imperative that *required* Bill Clinton to commit himself to comprehensive health care reform. This was a choice of conviction: He believes in it.

And so do those of us who threw ourselves into the reform effort. One day during the spring, as part of a series of meetings required of all the top policy staff, I was asked to spend an afternoon with about a dozen citizens who had written letters to Mrs. Clinton about their difficulties with the health care system. Their experiences were not unusual, though they spoke eloquently about them. Like millions of other Americans, they were facing big medical bills, struggling to take care of aging parents, trying to get insurers to cover preexisting conditions. They reminded us why we were there. Whether the policies we recommended were the right solutions to their problems, others will have to judge. But the interests we tried to serve, let no one doubt, were theirs.

PREFACE

One evening in early October 1991, I sat in a living room in a Philadelphia suburb talking about health insurance with Harris Wofford, whose name I had first heard only a few months before, when he was appointed to the U.S. Senate on the death of John Heinz. Now running against former Attorney General Richard Thornburgh for the rest of Heinz's term, Wofford was fighting his way up from a forty-point deficit in early polls. A few days earlier, his campaign manager James Carville had read an article of mine on the growing anxieties of the middle class about health insurance and called me to say that he and Wofford shared my analysis. Could I come down from Princeton to help the senator work through the issue? He had been making national health insurance the centerpiece of his campaign. By that October evening, with thiry-three days to go, the polls put him only twelve points behind.

Not everyone that fall thought campaigning on health insurance was a smart choice. E. J. Dionne of *The Washington Post* called health care "the issue from hell"—too complex and too costly to catch fire with the voters. One of the best informed researchers on public opinion and health care, Robert Blendon of the Harvard School of Public Health, told a reporter that health care was a "third-tier" political issue—way behind the economy, drugs, abortion, the budget deficit, and the savings and loan fiasco. Many once-ardent advocates of national health insurance had given up hope and either had quit trying to pass a program or were backing incremental changes. In the White House, President Bush was ignoring the issue.

But some analysts and politicians held a different view of the depth of discontent and the possibilities for comprehensive reform. For years, supporters of universal health insurance had framed it as an ethical challenge to help others in need; the problem, as they saw it, was how to spread to the poor one of the blessings enjoyed by the middle class. By the end of the 1980s, the issue had fundamentally changed. As health costs soared, businesses began to regard health benefits as an unmanageable burden: employers cut back benefits, insurance companies added preexisting condition exclusions and sought to screen out high-risk subscribers, and many in the middle class found that they had insecure protection. In their eyes, health insurance had changed from a problem that affects "them" to one that affects "us." That not only widened the potential constituency for reform; it also converted health insurance from a poverty issue into a general problem of economic prosperity. Wofford's upset landslide victory in Pennsylvania telegraphed the significance of that change to the country.

Yet three daunting obstacles stand in the way of action. The health care problem is genuinely complex; ideological conflict blocks any clear, consensus understanding; and the best organized interests in health care benefit from the present system because of the simplest equation of medical economics: *The costs of health care equal incomes from health care.* Rising costs have meant rising incomes; controlling costs means controlling incomes. The health care industry now represents a seventh of the U.S. economy, and the stakeholders in that industry—not just physicians, but hospitals, makers of medical equipment and pharmaceuticals, venture capitalists, and insurance companies—are not about to sit out a political battle that could so greatly affect their interests, in some cases their survival.

Earlier efforts to pass universal health insurance faced less daunting obstacles. National health insurance programs were introduced in Europe, Canada, and elsewhere when health care was a relatively minor industry and often before health insurance had had a chance to develop on a commercial basis. Governments bought off doctors by increasing their incomes. Indeed, despite their prior opposition, American doctors profited from the introduction of Medicare in 1965. Most likely they would also have gained, at least in the short term, from health insurance programs proposed in three earlier periods—before World War I, during the New Deal, and under the Truman administration. On sending his national health plan to Congress in 1945, President Truman noted that medical services "absorb only about 4 percent of the national income," and he declared, "We can afford to spend more for health." We could—and, in the years that followed, we did.

Sweetening the medicine of reform by paying doctors and hospitals more is no longer a political option. The imperatives have now changed, and universal access to health insurance is only part of what we need. The other part involves a fundamental reorganization of health care finance to ensure that costs grow at a controllable rate. Indeed, I favor universal health insurance not as a way to spend more money on health care: Properly designed, universal insurance offers the best chance and fairest method of curbing growth in the future, as it has done in the rest of the industrialized world.

Thus I see the problem in almost exactly the opposite

way from the conventional view. Most Americans wonder why we have not controlled health spending and how much more national health insurance might cost. I believe that we have not controlled costs because we lack the financial control that a comprehensive health insurance program produces.

Interest-based opposition to cost control may be enough, at least in the short run, to defeat any comprehensive health care reform. The ideological opposition makes the challenge even more formidable. From the earliest conflicts over government health insurance programs, the issue has evoked much sharper ideological differences in the United States than in Europe. European conservatives not only supported but often introduced national health insurance programs that American conservatives denounced as socialized medicine.

The debate in the United States has had a more inflammatory character, as opponents of publicly sponsored health insurance have typically sought to identify it with alien and subversive forces. The proposal died first in 1917–1918, when it was labeled an insidious German idea. It died a second time in the 1930s and '40s under a cloud of charges that the notion was Soviet-inspired. Lately, conservatives have condemned Canada's national health insurance as an alien, socialist scheme that individualistic Americans would never accept—even though Canada's health care providers are private, and Canadians choose freely among them.

The opposition between free choice and national health insurance is an old canard, but it is especially misleading today. The reality is that Americans are losing freedoms under the present system. Many people fear to change jobs because they would lose coverage of an existing health condition. That is a genuine loss of economic liberty. Many have been channeled by their employers into health plans that no longer allow them to go to their prior personal physician. And for the millions without insurance of any kind, "free choice" is a cruel way to describe their dependence on emergency rooms and exclusion from routine access to care. Universal coverage is itself a choice-expanding policy, and a good universal health insurance program can be designed, specifically for American circumstances, to increase the real options that we have.

Moreover, physicians, like consumers, have been losing freedom under the present system. The very failure to control costs in the United States has led both business and government to impose microregulation on health care that is more extensive than exists in countries with national health insurance. Many physicians from Europe, even from Great Britain, have commented that American doctors now face more paperwork, more regulations, and more second guessing of their decisions than is customary in countries where the government sets overall budgetary limits but leaves the detailed decisions about health care to the professionals. And as costs grow and insurance deteriorates, American doctors see more patients who cannot afford proper care and are postponing treatment of a health problem for fear of the expense. Increasingly, they feel that the health insurance system interferes with the practice of good medicine. So instead of insisting that no reform in health care finance is needed, many physicians have added their voices to those arguing on behalf of change—even fundamental change.

The approach to reform I take here attempts to enhance the liberty of consumers and providers as well as to meet the other great challenges of health policy: secure, equitable health coverage for all Americans, control of costs, high quality of care, and innovation.

The basic idea is not complicated: a public framework for insurance that allows Americans to choose among a variety of private health plans. But in America's highly polarized health care debate, the concept of a national health insurance program with competing private plans is exceptionally difficult to communicate. People immediately try to classify it on one or the other side of the ideological divide. If they hear "national" first, they identify it with a total government takeover. If they hear "competition" first, they identify it with the market approaches that reject the very idea of a common responsibility to ensure universal health coverage. Oversimplified media reports rarely get the idea straight.

The confusion has been aggravated by a mixup of the terms *managed care* and *managed competition*. Managed care describes a type—actually, several types—of health insurance plan. Managed competition refers to an approach to regulating the competition among plans, not all of which are based on managed care. Properly designed, managed competition would inhibit the growth of some managed care plans that now flourish only because they enroll healthier beneficiaries.

To add further to the confusion, managed competition refers to a way of organizing choices under both employment-based and publicly organized insurance programs. Some reports and editorials have specifically counterposed managed competition and national health insurance, as if the two were mutually exclusive. Yet in 1977, when Alain Enthoven first outlined a proposal for managed competition, it was presented and understood as an option for national health insurance.

In recent years, the phrase "national health insurance" has increasingly been identified with a federally financed and regulated insurance system—a more narrow conception than was current only a decade ago. When I use the phrase "national health insurance," I mean a system that provides access to a mainstream standard of coverage on the basis of citizenship rather than employment. All Americans would be included, and residents who are not citizens could qualify for coverage through their own or a family member's legal employment or study.

No proposal for health care reform can satisfy all the interests in health care, much less overcome the ideological divisions that exist between different groups and even within the medical profession. My aim is to cut through some of the fog that envelops the issue and foster a clearer understanding of the alternatives open to us today. National health policy is not a riddle without an answer. Unless we are ready to give up on the idea of self-government, surely we can do at least as well as the other major capitalist democracies in providing universal coverage, controlling costs, and satisfying public demands.

THE LOGIC OF HEALTH CARE REFORM

CHAPTER 1

A NEGATIVE CONSENSUS

It was a crisis. So said the news media. So said three quarters of the public, according to surveys. So said political leaders of both parties. All agreed that Americans faced a health care crisis created by "skyrocketing" costs, rampant inefficiency, and the continued lack of insurance coverage for millions of people. Seizing on the issue, liberal Democrats in Congress called for national health insurance; on the defensive, Republicans proposed more modest plans rooted in the private sector.

The year was 1971. A Rip Van Winkle who fell asleep then and awoke two decades later would have rubbed his eyes at a world transformed. Communism had collapsed in Eastern Europe, Germany was reunited, and the Soviet Union had disappeared from the map. But at least one thing would have been familiar: Americans were still fighting the same political battles over health care. The media were abuzz with talk of a health crisis, liberals called for national health insurance, and conservatives touted market-oriented alternatives.

Yet if our Rip Van Winkle began to ask what had happened over the two previous decades, he would soon discover that, despite appearances, the realities of health care in America had changed profoundly. Consider the following:

Since 1970 the economic stakes in the battle over health care have risen sharply. In 1970 *Business Week* called health care a "$60 billion crisis"; by 1993 health care was costing Americans $900 billion a year. Health care spending had risen from 7.3 percent to 14.3 percent of gross domestic product (GDP). Since 1981, health care has consumed an additional one percent of GDP *every 35 months.*

The trend of expanding health insurance coverage has been reversed. In the three decades before 1970, employer-based health plans and public programs covered an increasing proportion of Americans. But in the 1980s, coverage stopped expanding and the ranks of the uninsured began to grow.

Conventional health insurance was giving way to alternatives that often restricted consumers' choice of physicians and regulated physicians' choices of treatment. In 1970 most Americans had health insurance plans that reimbursed them for fee-for-service charges by whatever doctors and hospitals they chose and for virtually all recommended tests and treatments. By 1990 health maintenance organizations (HMOs) and other forms of managed care were becoming dominant, imposing restrictions that many doctors and patients would not have accepted two decades ago—such as requirements that patients consult a primary care physician before seeing a specialist and use designated hospitals, pharmacies, and other "in-network" facilities.

The health care industry has undergone other fundamental changes over the past two decades. The doctor shortage of the 1970s has turned into a glut in the 1990s—at least of specialists, who have poured onto the market in record numbers (even though in some communities primary care physicians continue to be relatively scarce). New types of ambulatory health centers and home health care businesses have proliferated, and many such services, as well as hospitals, are now owned and run by national chains. The provision of health care has changed in character from a traditional, low-key professional ethos to a more entrepreneurial, marketing orientation, aimed in part at stimulating new demands. Whole new medical technologies have arrived, the fruit of decades of biomedical research and an emerging revolution in biotechnology.

In a sense, the glut of specialists, the turn toward health care marketing, and the advent of new technologies are the fulfillment of policies adopted decades ago to spur medical research and education and the expansion of facilities. These policies have indeed produced some benefits originally hoped for. But from the standpoint of cost containment, they are like a time bomb detonating years after being planted, setting off serial explosions and side effects that no one foresaw.

Why Americans Want Change

Discontent with America's health care system is almost palpable. Polls now regularly find that 90 percent of Americans believe either that fundamental change is needed in health care or that the entire system has to be rebuilt. Employers are scarcely happy either. In a 1990 survey (conducted by Gallup for the Robert Wood Johnson Foundation), 91 percent of chief executive officers at Fortune 500 companies said that the system

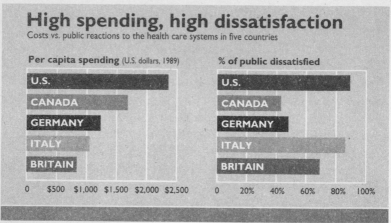

High spending, high dissatisfaction
Costs vs. public reactions to the health care systems in five countries

Per capita spending (U.S. dollars, 1989)

U.S.
CANADA
GERMANY
ITALY
BRITAIN

0    $500 $1,000 $1,500 $2,000 $2,500

% of public dissatisfied

U.S.
CANADA
GERMANY
ITALY
BRITAIN

0   20%   40%   60%   80%   100%

SOURCES: HARVARD-HARRIS-ITF TEN-NATION SURVEY, 1990; OECD

Among advanced societies, the U.S. ranks highest in both spending and dissatisfaction. People were "dissatisfied" if they said their system needs either "fundamental change" or to be "completely rebuilt."

needed fundamental change or a complete rebuilding.

These views amount to a negative consensus on the American health care system. Even the editor of the *Journal of the American Medical Association*, George D. Lundberg, declared in 1991 that fundamental reform had an air of "inevitability" about it. Like a city built on a geological fault, the health care system has been waiting for an earthquake. With President Clinton's election, the tectonic plates may have begun to move.

America's troubles with health care stand out sharply in international comparisons. A study that compared public opinion about health care in ten countries, conducted by Louis Harris and Associates in 1988 and 1990, found that the United States, along with Italy, had the highest level of public dissatisfaction with its health care system. Interestingly enough, public satisfaction in the ten countries was related to spending per capita: With lower spending generally came higher dissatisfaction (see chart, opposite page). The Italians' high dissatisfaction, for example, was in line with their country's extremely low per capita expenditures on health care. The one exception was the United States, which managed to have the lowest public approval while spending more for health care than any other country.

The exceptional pattern of health care spending in the United States is striking. While the U.S. is the one advanced industrialized country without national health insurance, other countries with national health insurance spend less. In 1991 (the latest year for which international data are available), the leading nations in Europe and North America, as well as Japan, spent an average of 7.9 percent of national income on health care. America's 13.2 percent that year was by far the highest. Per capita, the United States spent 40 percent more on health care than Canada, the second highest spender, and twice as much as major European nations. Year by year, the gap has been growing.

To be sure, surveys indicate that, while dissatisfied with the overall system, about three of every four Americans are satisfied with the quality of medical care they personally receive. Technically, American medicine is superb. What troubles the public, studies suggest, is the lack of secure insurance protection and uncontrolled health costs.

The usual measure of the insurance problem is the number of people who are without coverage at any one time—an estimated 38.9 million people in 1992, up 4.2 million from 1989. That represents more than one of six Americans under age sixty-five (17.4 percent), yet it understates the problem: In addition, some 40 million more Americans are estimated to be underinsured because their policies provide little protection in the event of serious illness. And according to a 1992 Census

Bureau study, one in four Americans (26 percent) had no health insurance coverage at some time over a twenty-eight-month period from 1987 to 1989.

Recessions in the United States not only increase job insecurity; they also make insecurity about health coverage pervasive since Americans in jeopardy of losing their jobs also worry about losing their health coverage. This linkage of insurance to jobs often doubles the loss and compounds the anxiety of unemployment. It is the peculiar evil of the American health insurance system that when the breadwinner of a family is thrown out of work, the entire family is threatened with loss of both secure access to health care and protection against financial devastation.

Yet the unemployed are only a minority of the uninsured. The majority of Americans without insurance are either working themselves or members of a family with an employed adult (see chart, opposite page). Typically they are the working poor, but many are middle class— or at least they used to be. During the 1980s, these people with jobs faced the biggest losses of coverage, as employers and health insurers tried to limit their own burdens and risks, often by cutting off coverage to people likely to incur high health care costs. This is an important new trend: Increasingly, Americans excluded from insurance protection are not just people with low incomes but middle class families with the misfortune of being hit with a potentially costly medical condition, like cancer, multiple sclerosis, or severe congenital problems in a newborn child.

The families of employees of small businesses and the self-employed have been in particular jeopardy of losing insurance (see chart). Many have faced staggering rate increases and are no longer able to afford insurance. Insurers have not only raised rates; they have "redlined"

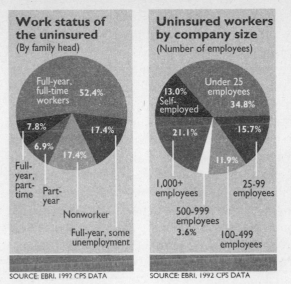

Work status of the uninsured
(By family head)

Full-year, full-time workers 52.4%

7.8%

17.4%

6.9%

17.4%

Full-year, part-time

Part-year

Nonworker

Full-year, some unemployment

Uninsured workers by company size
(Number of employees)

13.0% Self-employed

Under 25 employees 34.8%

21.1%

15.7%

11.9%

1,000+ employees

25-99 employees

500-999 employees 3.6%

100-499 employees

SOURCE: EBRI, 1992 CPS DATA

SOURCE: EBRI, 1992 CPS DATA

Over 38 million Americans under age sixty-five have no health insurance; more than 30 million of those are employed. About half of the uninsured who work are employed by companies with fewer than 100 employees.

entire industries and occupations, judging them to be "uninsurable." Some of these, like florists and hair stylists, are believed to be especially likely to include HIV-positive men, while others, such as sawmill workers, are considered prone to accidents. Some insurers have even blacklisted professional groups (including physicians!) because they tend to demand a lot of health care.

Many larger employers have also structured jobs and benefit plans to keep down the number of people they insure. It is no secret how companies avoid providing health benefits. They rely on part-time or short-term workers, or they contract out work to small firms that provide no benefits. Even some local governments have discovered they can save money by contracting out to private firms with uninsured workers. Some employers have also stopped paying for coverage of dependents. As a result, the percentage of children covered by employer-sponsored insurance has dropped sharply in the past decade. And when annually renewing their contracts with employers, some insurers have begun to exclude workers or dependents who have developed cancer and other high-cost conditions during the year.

This shrinkage of privately insured "risk pools" has been part of a general rollback of employer health benefits. In the face of annual premium increases averaging over 20 percent, employers have reduced their share of premiums, added deductibles and copayments, and switched to plans with more exclusions and limitations. Since 1980 the share of health premiums paid by employers has dropped from 80 percent to 69 percent. Many companies have also cut insurance coverage for their retirees, as the prospect of enormous liabilities has grown.

Another step, originally taken to cut insurance costs, has also heightened employees' insecurity about health coverage. Most large employers now "self-insure"—that is, they pay for the bills themselves, usually up to some stop-loss for which they do insure. Self-insurance allows employers to escape from state insurance regulations, including those mandating certain minimum levels of coverage. In 1991 a federal appeals court in New Orleans ruled in favor of a Texas company that self-insured and effectively terminated coverage of AIDS-related illnesses when costs for an employee suffering from the disease soared. According to the court, employers that self-insure are not legally obligated to maintain coverage. They can terminate it at any time—and some are doing just that.

In addition, some insurance companies have simply cancelled coverage when policyholders have submitted large claims, or they have refused payment on the grounds that the subscribers must have withheld information on the original insurance application. Because of lax insurance regulation, says a study by the U.S. General Accounting Office (GAO), some 400,000 Americans were left uninsured between 1988 and 1990 when their insurers folded up operations. Many more workers have been stranded when their companies disappeared in bankruptcies and mergers.

Another development that adds to the public's feeling of insecurity is the growing number of health plans that exclude coverage of preexisting medical conditions. The majority of employers who offer insurance today have policies with such exclusions. Some plans, in fact, do not merely exclude specific conditions; they deny any coverage to individuals if they have had one of a list of serious conditions at some time in the past. Unknown fifteen years ago, such clauses can have devastating effects. A child born disabled loses health coverage when a parent changes jobs. A woman whose cancer has been in remission learns that she has no insurance coverage when another tumor is discovered after her husband has changed employers. Under current statutes such exclusions are entirely legal.

Preexisting condition clauses not only deny millions of Americans health coverage when they most need it; such clauses also limit opportunities for economic mobility. Many employees now hesitate to change jobs for fear of losing coverage. In a 1991 *New York Times*–CBS poll, three of ten Americans said they or someone in their household has experienced this kind of job lock. And when people are deprived of opportunities for job mobility, the economy is deprived of potentially greater contributions they could make elsewhere—an indirect and unmeasured cost of our health care system.

Insecurity about health coverage thus involves several distinct concerns. Americans are not only worried about the risk of being uninsured; even those who are insured are worried about being denied coverage when the real need comes and of being tied down to a particular job, slaves to health insurance. The spread of exclusions and limitations, arbitrary terminations of coverage, and outright fraud are some of the reasons why Rashi Fein, an economist at Harvard, says that health insurance in America might be better called "unsurance."

Many Americans are deeply angry about being stuck with "unsurance"; they feel abandoned and betrayed. They've worked hard for years on the assumption that they would receive certain things in return, one of them being health benefits. When they lose that protection, they see everything they have built in jeopardy.

Perhaps most disturbing, they know that all the trends affecting insurance coverage have been moving in the wrong direction. A 1991 survey of small employers by Louis Harris found that 13 percent had recently eliminated health insurance benefits and another 30 percent expect to be forced to drop them in the future. As health coverage evaporates, employees ask themselves how they will be able to hang on to their standard of living. Americans today do not have to be poor to worry that the country's system for financing health care will someday impoverish them.

Why America Needs Change

The costs and insecurities felt directly by the public are grounds enough for reform, but the health care problem has still wider dimensions. The system's costs and indirect effects are key factors in the deeper fiscal and economic problems besetting the United States.

The health costs that hit most Americans directly—increased employee contributions for insurance premiums and growing out-of-pocket expenses for copayments, deductibles, and uncovered services—are only the tip of the health cost iceberg. Employees generally do not know how much their employer pays for their health insurance; few understand how large a tax subsidy they enjoy because an employer's contributions do not count toward their own taxable income. Even fewer people have any idea what share of their taxes goes to health care. If anything, public perceptions are structurally biased to underestimate health care costs. In a sense, public dissatisfaction with health costs is all the more compelling because Americans have been cushioned against the full burden.

For both business and government, the rising cost of health care has become a chronic economic ailment. Between 1948 and 1990, business spending on health benefits has grown an average of 15.6 percent a year, climbing to more than 8 percent of payroll (wages and salaries). Most economists argue that the higher cost of health benefits has not reduced profits; they maintain—with strong supporting evidence—that the costs have come out of workers' pay instead. The majority of people are unlikely to find comfort in that conclusion. Since the early 1970s, real take-home pay has stagnated, in part because health benefits have absorbed over half the increases in compensation. And notwithstanding the general rule that workers ultimately bear the costs, many firms are convinced that the high cost of health insurance has been hurting their profitability,

Rise in employer spending 1970–1989

Per full-time employee

175%
150%
125%
100%
75%
50%
25%
0

Wages and salaries

Retirement benefits

Other fringe benefits

Health benefits

SOURCE: ALLIANCE FOR HEALTH REFORM, EBRI DATA

Employers' spending on health benefits has risen far more rapidly than other forms of employee compensation. Measured in constant 1989 dollars, this category increased 163 percent between 1970 and 1989.

which is why they have changed and cut back their benefit plans.

The impact on the public sector has been just as serious. Government costs for health care have risen at 11 percent a year, three to four times above recent inflation. Because of slow economic growth and wide resistance to higher taxes, increased health costs have necessarily cut into other public programs. In effect, health care has crowded out other needs from the public budget.

The shift of public expenditures to health care may harm not only other social needs but also economic growth. Over the past several decades, the portion of public spending devoted to investment has declined sharply. Investment in roads, bridges, and other additions to the stock of public wealth commanded 6.9 percent of public spending between 1945 and 1952 but only 1.2 percent in the 1980s. Public investments have a payoff in the future; borrowing for purposes of investment has a sound economic logic. But while federal borrowing has hit record levels in the past decade, the United States has shifted public spending from investment to consumption—of which most health spending is a prime example.

The crowding out of productive public investment is one of several ways in which the growth of the health care system now impinges on the nation's productivity. I have already mentioned the reduction of job mobility. While the insurance system locks some Americans in their current jobs, it locks others into welfare. The principal alternative to welfare lies in low-paying jobs that typically do not carry health benefits. Since moving off welfare often means losing Medicaid, millions on welfare find that if they work they cannot have secure access to health care. One major benefit of universal health insurance would be to promote the transition of the dependent from welfare to work.

In addition, health benefits have become a major source of friction between labor and management. In recent years, according to the AFL-CIO, the scaling back of health benefits has been the cause of the majority of strikes in the United States. That too is a cost of our insurance system which countries with national health insurance do not face.

Few deny that health care in America is too costly, but some are curiously indifferent to it. What percentage of GDP, they ask, is the right percentage to spend on health care anyway? Isn't our spending for health care creating new jobs? And isn't it a natural, evolutionary shift in a postindustrial, service economy to spend a rising share of GDP on health care?

In the 1950s and '60s, when we were in the early stages of the health sector's expansion, these were reasonable thoughts. But as costs in the U.S. have risen farther from the average in other advanced societies, it has become clear that a peculiar dynamic is at work in the United States, eroding real wages and the fiscal integrity of government. One comparison particularly helps to bring the rise of spending for health care into sharp relief. In 1965 the United States spent about the same percentage of GDP on each of three sectors—education (6.2 percent), health care (5.9 per-

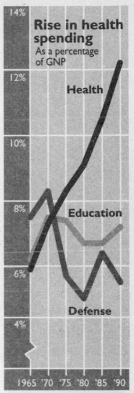

Rise in health spending
As a percentage of GNP

Health

Education

Defense

1965 '70 '75 '80 '85 '90

SOURCES: HCFA, NATIONAL CENTER FOR EDUCATION STATISTICS, STATISTICAL ABSTRACT OF THE U.S.

The U.S. currently spends about twice as much on health care as it does on education or national defense. In the early '70s, the three sectors consumed approximately equal portions of the GNP.

cent), and defense (7.5 percent). The military's share has now fallen beneath 6 percent and is projected to drop farther during the 1990s, while education has edged up slightly, to 7.2 percent. But the share spent on health care has more than doubled, to 14.3 percent. Projections by the Clinton administration and Congressional Budget Office suggest it may reach between 17.5 percent and 18 percent by the year 2000. This vast shift of national resources is proceeding without any clear understanding or public discussion of its long-term adverse repercussions for the country.

And despite this fantastic rate of spending, there is the ultimate irony: We do not have a healthier society than do other Western countries that spend far less. This ought not to be surprising. Studies have long shown that spending on health care is not a major determinant of a nation's health. Yet without reform of the nation's health care financing system, there is no way to shift resources toward uses that would be genuinely conducive to health as well as prosperity.

Back in 1971, when our Rip Van Winkle nodded off, there was an abundance of fresh ideas about reforming the health care system. While there was a sense of crisis, there was also a sense of optimism about possible remedies. Since then, many of those remedies have been tried without success. Now there is a readiness to go beyond mere tinkering but nowhere agreed upon to go. From the negative consensus about the status quo, Americans have not yet been able to fashion a positive consensus about an alternative. And that, in part, is because we have no clear understanding of where and why the system is failing.

C H A P T E R   2

WHAT WENT WRONG?

Among the many explanations for America's continuing crisis of health care costs, two lines of thought stand out. One view traces rising costs to many different "cost drivers," prominently including Americans' high expectations and demands, new technologies, malpractice litigation, and the aging of the population. This approach often produces long laundry lists of recommendations for piecemeal reforms. It also encourages the perception that we are all responsible for the problems of health care and, perhaps, that no one is really responsible because high costs reflect cultural patterns and demographic trends beyond anyone's control. It is a view endorsed by much of the leadership of the health care industry.

A second line of explanation emphasizes health care finance and organization. While acknowledging that ingrained cultural attitudes, technological change, and aging have had some effect on costs, this approach focuses on the economic structure of the system as the key cause of America's rising costs and deteriorating insurance coverage.

I am an advocate of this systemic interpretation and, hence, of systemic reform. But before laying out that view, or at least one version of it, I want to take on the explanations that constitute the conventional wisdom and that provide a consoling vision of the health cost problem.

Consoling Explanations

Consoling Explanation No. 1: Americans expect more. It is a comforting and even flattering thought that we have higher medical costs because Americans are especially demanding and have higher expectations than do people elsewhere. It suggests we have more sophistication and more rigorous standards than foreigners who accept "nationalized" health care. This argument also implicitly warns against systemic changes that would require us to lower our expectations.

But is it true that American patients are more demanding and that these higher demands cause our higher costs? The health care decision affecting costs that is most under the control of consumers is the initial choice to contact a doctor. If Americans really are especially demanding, we should expect them to consult physicians more frequently than do people elsewhere. Yet the annual rate of physician visits in the United States is below average for industrialized countries. In fact, the American rate of 5.5 visits per year is less than half that of Germany (11.5 visits) and Japan (12.9 visits), both of which have lower health care costs (see chart, page 18).

This should not be surprising. The costs of health care systems in advanced societies are not concentrated at the front end, where consumers have most control over the care they receive. Rather, costs are concentrated later on, typically in a hospital, where doctors and health care managers have most control. This pattern suggests that the incentives and constraints influencing their decisions are crucial.

The argument that Americans' high demands cause high costs assumes that high costs in the U.S. reflect a higher level of service. Compared to health care in other industrialized countries, America's system certainly does provide far more cardiac surgery and organ transplants, although less primary and preventive care. But the spending gap between the U.S. and other countries is not due primarily to the high rate of high-tech care in the U.S.

The most detailed comparisons of American with foreign health expenditures have involved Canada, which, as we have seen, is the world's second highest spender. Of the Canadian–U.S. expenditure difference (now amounting to about 4 percent of GNP), between a third and a half is due to higher administrative and insurance costs in the United States. Roughly another third reflects the higher expense of physicians' services. A carefully controlled comparison of expenditures for physicians' services in the two countries showed, however, that in 1985 and 1987 Canadians, while spending less, actually received a higher volume of physicians' services. The difference in cost was entirely explained by higher physician fees in the U.S. (The U.S. does spend more for medical research, accounting for a small percentage of the total difference with Canada.)

Finally, the remaining gap reflects higher costs for hospital care in the United States. According to a comparative study of Canadian and American hospitals, admission rates are about the same, while stays are longer

How America stacks up internationally

	Health spending* per capita	Inpatient days per capita	Physician contacts per capita	Infant mortality per 1,000 live births	Life expectancy (male)		Percent of population age 65 and over
					at birth	at age 80	
U.S.	$2,868	1.2	5.5	9.1	72.0	7.1	12.3
CANADA	$1,915	2.0	6.9	6.8	73.8	7.1	11.1
GERMANY	$1,659	3.3	11.5	7.1	72.6	6.1	15.4
JAPAN	$1,307	4.1	12.9	4.6	75.9	6.9	11.2
BRITAIN	$1,043	2.0	5.7	7.9	73.0	6.2	15.6
OECD average for 24 nations	$1,305	2.7	6.2	9.7	72.6	6.4	13.0

* In U.S. dollars, 1991

SOURCE: *HEALTH AFFAIRS*, FALL 1991 AND SUMMER 1993; OECD DATA

Although the U.S. spends more for health care than any other nation, international comparisons indicate that its citizens do not necessarily receive better care than do residents of nations that spend less.

in Canada. American hospital care, however, is far more costly because of what happens after admission. Costs run 50 percent greater in U.S. hospitals because the hospitals use more "inputs" (that is, they do more tests, procedures, and so on) and because the hospitals pay more for their inputs. One cause may be the much greater share of American nurses' time consumed by filling out forms required for reimbursement and regulation, which not only raises costs but interferes with personal care.

Consumers hardly desire higher administrative and insurance costs or higher physician and hospital prices, but what about the greater intensiveness of medical care? That American medicine is more procedure-oriented and technologically intensive is a routine finding of comparative health care research. Some analysts point to an aggressive therapeutic style evident, for example, in more radical surgical interventions favored by doctors in the United States when compared, for example, with their French and British peers. These differences in practice style seem to reflect patterns of medical training in the U.S, the much higher rate of specialization among American physicians, and the financial incentives for both doctors and hospitals to emphasize procedures.

Some patients in the United States are sufficiently well informed to expect and demand a lot of specific tests and procedures, and they might well be dissatisfied with the technology available at community hospitals in most other Western countries. One study, conducted for the Robert Wood Johnson Foundation, finds that a much higher percentage of Americans than of foreigners say they would seek a second opinion if their physician said they had a terminal illness. Americans who are denied experimental treatments sometimes go on radio and television to plead for public support—a phenomenon not seen elsewhere.

Still, it is hard to see how patients could have shaped the prevailing patterns of medical practice and hospital management. Most patients leave choice of treatment to their doctors; physicians and other professionals educate the public about appropriate styles of care. In explaining differences in technological intensiveness, the direction of causality seems at least as likely to run from the health care system to public attitudes as from public attitudes to the system.

Consoling Explanation No. 2: Malpractice litigation. Many people, especially physicians, are convinced that high malpractice insurance rates and the practice of defensive medicine to avoid suits are major sources of excessive health costs in the United States. Once again, the

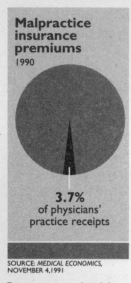

Malpractice insurance premiums
1990

3.7%
of physicians'
practice receipts

SOURCE: MEDICAL ECONOMICS,
NOVEMBER 4, 1991

On average, physicians pay less than 4 percent of annual practice receipts for malpractice insurance. That amounts to less than 1 percent of total U.S. health expenditures.

claim is that Americans are different—more litigious as patients and more likely as jurors to give big verdicts for plaintiffs.

Yet the evidence does not bear out the hypothesis that malpractice litigation is a major source of the cost problem.

Since malpractice insurance represents less than 1 percent of overall health costs, it cannot possibly be a primary cause of the growth in expenditures. To be sure, some medical specialties in some states have faced staggering rate increases. These periodic shocks reflect the cyclical nature of the insurance business and the inability of insurers to spread risks beyond the members of one specialty in one state. Overall, malpractice insurance premiums have been virtually constant as a share of physician costs.

The impact of defensive medicine on costs is more difficult to evaluate. Although some procedures adopted defensively are unnecessary, others represent legitimate quality assurance. There are no good estimates of the cost of the truly unnecessary procedures. We also do not know how many patients avoid medical injuries because of defensively adopted procedures. Some precautions that seem unnecessary may turn out to prevent mistakes. Thus the *net* economic impact of defensive medicine is unclear.

Furthermore, doctors and hospitals generally make money off the procedures that they perform, even if they do them defensively. Stanford health economist Victor Fuchs has asked the pointed, hypothetical question: "If new legislation outlawed all future malpractice claims, by how much would physicians and hospitals voluntarily cut their present revenues?" Anyone who thinks that defensive medicine is a big problem must believe that providers would sacrifice billions of dollars in revenues. This seems highly implausible.

Some reforms of malpractice law, such as arbitration procedures to settle cases out of court, do make sense. The tort system is neither an efficient nor effective way to raise the quality of care. Research has shown that most medical negligence is never even brought to court. And only a small portion of the money paid out in malpractice premiums ends up compensating plaintiffs (the great bulk being consumed by insurance companies and lawyers). Yet as sensible as reforms may be, not even the most extensive changes in the malpractice system are likely to alter the general trend in health care costs.

Consoling Explanation No. 3: Aging. There is no question that it costs more on average to care for the aged than for younger people and that the proportion of the aged in the population is slowly but appreciably growing. Those realities give rise to a genuine long-term problem, which will be especially acute once the baby boom generation reaches advanced old age.

But thus far, aging has been only a secondary factor in overall health sector expansion. The share of GDP devoted to health spending has not soared in recent decades because of a massive onset of old age. According to one estimate, aging alone caused a 0.3 percent annual increase in the use of health services over the forty years prior to 1986. Moreover, age differences do not help account for international differences in health spending. The reason the U.S. spends more on health than do other countries is not that it has a larger elderly population. Among twenty-four industrialized nations, the U.S. ranks seventeenth in the percentage of population age sixty-five or over. In particular, the Scandinavian countries, Germany, and Britain have much larger elderly populations—about 25 percent greater relative to the U.S. As these examples illustrate, how many elderly people a country has is less important than how it manages and pays for the health care of all age groups. The U.S. system generates high costs for all Americans, and especially high costs for care of the aged, making the aged not the cause but a key focus of the problem.

Health care costs did rise more rapidly for the aged after the introduction of Medicare; what is more surprising is that they have continued to rise disproportionately in recent years. The remedy, however, lies less in special rules for care of the aged than in general reform of the system. Perhaps what should disturb us most is that we have already seen a vast increase in health care costs *before* the big demographic shift toward the aged that is expected in the next century.

Consoling Explanation No. 4: Technology. Those who argue that new technology is the primary cause of higher costs generally have in mind big-ticket items such as new imaging technologies, organ transplantation, intensive care units, and renal dialysis. Such innovations have undoubtedly brought higher costs, but as we have seen, only about a third of the higher levels of U.S. spending, compared with Canada, reflects the greater expense of hospital care—and of that, only a portion is due to greater use of technology.

Certainly, there are differences in technology. For example, the U.S. has eight times more magnetic resonance imaging (MRI) facilities than does Canada on a per capita basis, and we do twenty-six times as much heart bypass surgery as do some major European countries.

But do our higher levels reflect appropriate use and sound decisions about investment? While waiting lists in Canada may reveal organizational inefficiencies and insufficient levels of investment (depending on how urgent the procedures genuinely are), many high-tech services in the United States have been overbuilt and then used for purposes for which they have never been demonstrated to be effective. For example, computerized tomography (CT scanning) radically improved treatment of head injuries but was then misused to investigate headaches.

At the core of the problem is the relationship between doctors and hospitals. Hospitals do not sell their services directly but only through physicians, who are free to take their patients and purchasing power elsewhere. (Increasingly, physicians themselves have set up independent imaging centers and other facilities to participate directly in the profits.) To keep their beds filled, hospitals must keep their doctors happy. They duplicate costly technologies and then use them well below capacity because institutional imperatives overwhelmingly press them to do so.

In other markets, excess supply drives down prices; the supplier who refuses to cut prices loses customers and may go out of business. Why doesn't that happen in health care? The answer brings us to the heart of the matter: the perverse and peculiar features of health care markets.

The Systemic View

The American health care system has developed under the shaping influence of incentives for private decision makers to expand and intensify medical services. These incentives are now entrenched in the system's physical structures and everyday practices. Their effects have been magnified by public policies adopted between the 1940s and '60s that generated more doctors, more hospital capacity, and more technology. Then, when government and business tried to control costs, they found they had denied themselves the instruments necessary to do so.

Traditional insurance for fee-for-service medical care lacks any of the usual checks on consumption. When buying a house or a hamburger, consumers usually have to weigh the costs against other possible expenditures. They also can, and do, compare the price and value of what various sellers are offering. Under third-party health insurance, however, patients have little incentive to weigh costs carefully, and because they lack sufficient knowledge they generally rely on professionals for guidance on treatment and other critical decisions affecting costs. With some exceptions, the professionals who make the decisions can increase their earnings by providing more services. It is no surprise, therefore, that many of them do so. Moreover, the fragmentation and complexity of the system generate an administrative burden of staggering dimensions.

These incentives have literally been built into the health care system. They have guided investment decisions about the construction of hospitals and purchase of equipment. They have influenced young doctors' choices of specialty: We have too many surgeons and too few primary care doctors because our financing system has for decades encouraged doctors to invest in surgical training. These incentives, moreover, have influenced the everyday rules of thumb that doctors use in deciding about tests, hospitalization, operations, and so on. The practice styles of American physicians are partly the product of financial arrangements that for decades rewarded the decision to treat even if there was no good evidence the treatment would work. In short, financial incentives have become entrenched in physical assets, the distribution of specialists, and the patterns of accepted medical practice.

This result is not just incidental waste and a few flagrant abuses but a vast misallocation of resources. In the conventional fee-for-service sector, Americans experience about 960 days of hospital care per thousand persons; in prepaid group practice plans, the comparable figure is 460 days. Studies evaluating the appropriateness of care indicate that as much as 30 percent of the surgery performed in the United States is unnecessary. Taking all the sources of inefficiency together, Arnold Relman, the former editor of *The New England Journal of Medicine*, estimates that roughly one third of health care expenditures are medically unnecessary.

The distortions of investment in health care resources are not only costly; they also reduce our capacity to provide good medical care. With too many specialists but not enough primary care physicians, we have much unnecessary surgery but too little immunization of children. With too great a supply of imaging technology, used at too low a rate, hospitals and clinics raise prices to recoup their investment, and the services become inaccessible to many who might benefit from them.

Consider the case of early detection of breast cancer through the use of mammography. With fully utilized mammography machines, a screening mammography examination should cost no more than $55, according to studies by the GAO and Physician Payment Review Commission. But because machines are typically used far beneath capacity, prices run double that amount. With prices so high, many women cannot afford a mammogram (indeed, at such high prices, it is not clear that mammography can survive a stringent cost-benefit test).

In other words, *because we have too many mammography machines, we have too little breast cancer screening.* Only in America are poor women denied a mammogram because there is too much equipment.

This is symptomatic of the larger problem: The public health failures of the American medical system are not the result of our spending too little; they often stem from spending too much the wrong way, thereby producing patterns of practice and organization ill suited to primary care, prevention, and public health.

Of course, we cannot undo the past choices that have given us our present system. But we can at least begin changing the legacy that we leave to the next generation by shifting incentives away from overspecialization, overbuilding, and overspending. To do so, we need to change health care finance systemically—that, in fact, is the great opportunity of national health reform.

C H A P T E R 3

HOPE AMID THE RUINS

Uncontrolled growth in costs and deepening insecurities about insurance are not only problems in health care; they are also an index of political failure. How to respond to rising health costs has been a major concern of national policy for the past twenty years; and for even longer, reformers have sought to extend insurance coverage to the entire population. Both business and government have launched countless programs attacking one or another part of the problem. There has been no shortage of research to evaluate alternative approaches. But political deadlock has prevented any fundamental breakthrough.

This paralysis has created a dangerous sense of frustration and despair. Many have concluded that the problem of health spending is intractable and that there is no way to cover all of the uninsured without making things worse. Unable to control costs through minor adjustments of policy, some in Congress and state legislatures ultimately see no alternative but to adopt a system for rationing medical care (that is, consciously limiting beneficial care by administrative priorities). After all, if high expectations are responsible for our costs, we must lower them; if technological advance is responsible, we must slow it; if aging is responsible, we must set some arbitrary age limit on treatment—or so it would seem to many who hold the conventional view. Thus does a harsh realism spring from the frustrations of reform.

Yet there is, as I have suggested, an alternative view. The 14 percent of GDP we spend on health care should be more than enough to provide universal coverage and a high quality of care. But to keep spending under control requires a strategy for structural change to reverse the entrenched patterns of investment and behavior that will threaten the solvency of any program for universal coverage. And to figure out such a strategy, we need to understand why reform measures have thus far failed and where, amid the ruins of policy, we can find the sources of hope and reconstruction.

The Failure of Halfway Reform

At first appearance, the single best argument for believing that cost control must end in rationing is that the steps taken so far to control costs have not worked. But the reasons for that failure do not suggest that the problem is insurmountable, only that we have not addressed it coherently. While some public policies have attempted to restrain costs, others have been powerfully promoting their growth, and the most important structural forces behind the cost explosion have remained unchecked.

Early efforts to control costs, rather than altering the organization of medical practice and hospitals, created a second level of review above them. In the 1970s, the federal government and the states initiated two major regulatory efforts: utilization review, to check up on physicians' and hospitals' treatment and billing, and health care planning agencies, to review hospitals' capital investment decisions. Utilization review programs retrospectively examined the paper trail of clinical decisions; consequently, reviewers were remote from the clinical scene and had no capacity to ask for new clinical data or to encourage a more cost-effective approach in particular cases. They could do nothing but deny payment afterward. The programs challenged exceptional cases of excessive cost or doubtful quality, while accepting the routine but inefficient practices that are the crux of the problem.

Similarly, the planning agencies were entirely reactive, their authority primarily negative. They advised state governments on whether or not to approve hospital expansion plans but they had little creative, shaping power—indeed, no power at all—to limit or redirect capital investment to get better value for money. Like utilization review programs, the health planning agencies sought, in practice, to curb the worst excesses of the system; they did not challenge its standard operating procedures.

Both utilization review and health planning were weak brakes applied to a vehicle being driven with the accelerator to the floor. Under fee-for-service payment, doctors profit the more services they provide. Medicare, like Blue Cross, imposed no fee schedule: Doctors were assured payment if the fees they demanded were "usual, customary, and reasonable." Cost-based reimbursement to hospitals invited hospitals to run up costs. These were arrangements that the doctors and hospitals had secured through effective lobbying. From the beginning, they were a recipe for fiscal disaster.

One regulatory effort dating from the early 1970s had

some modest success in restraining costs, but its limitations are also instructive. A handful of states, including Maryland, New Jersey, and New York, regulated hospital prices and succeeded in holding down the rate of growth in hospital expenditures somewhat beneath the national average. But hospital costs are a function of three factors: volume, price, and the intensity of services. Rate setting can slow price increases without controlling the other sources of growth. In addition, rate setting, like health planning, applied exclusively to hospitals. Thus it invited a shift of technology and services from hospitals into ambulatory care centers and doctors' offices to escape regulatory control.

With the 1979 congressional defeat of federal hospital cost containment legislation proposed by President Carter, regulatory efforts to control overall hospital costs reached a dead end, at least for a time. In the 1980s, with the advent of the Reagan administration, the emphasis in health policy was supposed to shift from regulation to competition. At the outset of the Reagan years, several models of market-oriented reform, including a bill introduced in 1978 by Representatives David Stockman and Richard Gephardt (an odd couple, in retrospect), were circulating in Washington. Among other things, pro-competitive reform called for changes in tax policy to make employees more sensitive to health insurance costs, a broad attack on monopolistic practices in the health professions, and strong support for HMOs and other alternative health plans. But a comprehensive, pro-competitive approach to health care turned out to lack support even among Republicans, and the administration abandoned the effort. Instead, Congress enacted measures to make the federal government a more "prudent buyer" of health care and thereby limit the costs of federal programs.

The most important initiative was the new hospital payment system that Congress adopted in 1983 to replace Medicare's previous arrangement for reimbursing hospitals. Hospitals would now be paid per admission, rather than per day and per service. Reimbursement rates, divided into some 470 diagnosis-related groups (DRGs), would be set in advance, thus putting hospitals at risk (if costs exceeded the prospective payment, it was their loss; if costs were lower, their gain). For the first time, hospitals were given a strong incentive to control costs through such measures as discharge planning.

Yet the DRG system provides no incentive to reduce unnecessary admissions; and since it affects hospitals but not doctors, it gives doctors no incentives for cost containment. Moreover, Medicare's payment system does not apply to other payers, onto which hospitals can, and do, shift unreimbursed costs. As a result, hospitals have continued to be profitable even at astonishingly low occupancy rates.

The federal government has also moved to reform physician payment. From its outset, Medicare reproduced and reinforced the incentives favoring "procedural" over "cognitive" services (for example, surgery over medical consultations) and urban over rural physicians, thereby helping to distort the specialty and geographical distribution of physicians. The resource-based relative value scale, the key element in the reformed payment system, ranks physician services according to the complexity of tasks and the resources they consume. Ideally, the new approach should counteract the longstanding biases in physician payment; in practice, because of concessions to specialists, its effects are likely to be modest.

These steps toward payment reform, while generally positive, have simply not been enough: They have been slow in coming, compromised in execution, and limited in effect because of the ability of hospitals and doctors to shift costs to the private sector. When hospital costs are controlled, providers shift services to the ambulatory side. When the government acts to discipline costs, providers typically charge more to the privately insured. Lacking any comprehensive mechanism of control, payers have been at a sharp disadvantage in their cost containment battles with providers.

Employers, like the federal government, have revised their health benefit plans to limit costs. In addition to self-insuring, many have required employees to share a higher proportion of costs at the time of illness. Cost-sharing does tend to reduce demand, but it has serious drawbacks. Patients appear to cut down as much on needed as on unneeded contacts with physicians, and cost-sharing does little to reduce the costs associated with the most expensive phases of care in the hospital, where patients exercise little control. Employers adopted other measures to control these costs. Some paid for, or even required, second opinions prior to surgery. Some contracted with outside firms for case management to control the use of services, imposing requirements such as pre-admission certification for hospitalization. In recent years, many companies have moved toward managed care as a comprehensive solution. Although the picture here is more complicated—and I shall have more to say about it in a moment—these efforts have thus far brought no general slowing of national health expenditures.

Once facilities, technology, and manpower are in place, it is hard for any one payer, governmental or private, to do much but shift costs elsewhere. The decisions that most affect how much it costs to operate the health care system are the "upstream" choices about what kind of system to have in the first place: investment decisions about the physical capacity of the system, its technological complexity, and the specialized training of its key decision makers, physicians. Because of the inherent uncertainty and ambiguity of medical decisions, physicians can easily prescribe more services to fit available time and budgets. If there are more physicians, they will find more to do—more tests to run, more need for surgery, more patients requiring followup. Economists call this "supplier induced demand." While the extra services provided may individually seem reasonable, they have little impact on a society's overall health.

Throughout this period of halfway regulation in the 1970s and '80s—"halfway" because the basic incentives for increasingly costly health services were left in place—the supply of physicians, and particularly of specialists, was rising rapidly (see chart, right). Federal policies affecting physician training adopted in the 1960s more than doubled the number of medical school graduates, and these graduates overwhelmingly became subspecialists. Investment in hospitals and high-tech services grew rapidly, stimulated in part by generous provisions in Medicare for reimbursing hospitals' capital costs. Whatever might have been accomplished by regulation was undone by these other developments.

The regulatory programs were destined to fail because

Rise in supply of U.S. physicians

Physicians per 100,000 population

300
250
225
200
175
150
125

1960 '65 '70 '75 '80 '85 '90

SOURCES: AMERICAN MEDICAL ASSOCIATION; U.S. CENSUS DATA

The number of doctors has grown far faster than the U.S. population for three decades. There are now 72 percent more physicians per 100,000 Americans than in 1960.

they never imposed firm ceilings on investment or expenditures, nor changed the underlying incentives facing providers and patients, nor required institutions to match their resources to the needs of the populations they served. In the United States the matching of resources to the needs of populations happened only in one significant arena: health maintenance organizations. And yet here too reform failed to produce the general revolution in health care that business and government were seeking.

The Rise of HMOs

In the early 1970s, enthusiasm developed among politicians and health care policy makers for home-grown health care organizations long described as "prepaid group practices" or "group health plans." The early group health plans, such as the Kaiser Foundation Health Plan and Group Health Cooperative of Puget Sound, were founded in the 1930s and '40s to provide comprehensive, high-quality medical care primarily to employee groups. Almost accidentally, the plans turned out to reduce the overall costs of health care compared to conventional, fee-for-service health insurance.

Reports in the 1950s and '60s that the plans produced substantial savings set off a long and bitter debate. Many critics, especially private physicians, insisted that group health plans had lower costs only because they provided shoddy service, their enrollees were healthier, and members were getting additional services outside the plans. Besides, they said, most Americans are too individualistic and too demanding to accept the "compromises" of a socialistic, group plan. It took a lot of expensive research to show that the plans' savings were genuine, ranging from 10 to 40 percent, as compared to fee-for-service care under conventional insurance plans.

The reduced costs chiefly reflected a drastically reduced rate of hospital use. In what is generally regarded as the most reliable randomly controlled study, the RAND Corporation's health insurance experiment in Seattle (conducted from 1976 to 1980) found savings of 28 percent from prepaid group practice, with no adverse effects on health outcomes. Numerous other studies have also demonstrated that prepaid group-practice plans provide medical care of at least equal quality as fee-for-service medicine.

Yet prepaid group practices are not easy to start. They require the development of multispecialty medical groups and special managerial skills, both of which are relatively scarce. Furthermore, as of the early 1970s, more than thirty states had laws that effectively barred prepaid group-practice plans, and most businesses did not offer them to their employees.

Searching for a distinct approach to health care, the Nixon administration in 1970 became the first to make the development of prepaid plans a central element in national health policy. The impetus came from Paul Ellwood, a Minnesota pediatric neurologist who coined the term *health maintenance organization*. (As a specialist in rehabilitation, Ellwood had become convinced that prepayment made more sense than fee-for-service.) The HMO concept included not only the prepaid group-practice plans but also a variant, "independent practice associations" (IPAs), which were more acceptable to fee-for-service practitioners.

A peculiar feature of IPAs is that they present one face to the consumer, another to the physician. They charge capitation (per person) rates to subscribers or their employers but provide care through doctors in private practice whom they generally pay by fee-for-service, although at a discount from their usual rates. The difference is often withheld in a fund for profit sharing at year's end. Compared to prepaid group-practice plans, IPAs are less costly to launch, and they do not necessarily require patients to give up their family physician. At least until recently, they have not shown many of the organizational capacities of the group-practice plans for assuring quality and promoting more efficient patterns of practice. However, some plans based on networks of independent physicians have been developing in that direction.

As HMOs evolved over the past two decades, further varieties have emerged. Some IPAs rely on a primary care physician to control referrals and hospitalization. These doctors are known as gatekeepers and are sometimes paid by capitation rather than fee-for-service. While financial arrangements vary, plans that offer doctors incentives to control referrals may create a conflict between physicians' pocketbook interests and decisions about additional patient care. Such ethical dilemmas, however, are scarcely unknown in the fee-for-service sector, since a family practitioner may worry that a patient referred to a specialist may never come back.

With the inclusion of IPAs and gatekeeper plans, the original idea of prepaid group practice changed dramatically. The early organizations began with a commitment to comprehensive care and incidentally turned out to have lower costs. The new organizations were created to cut costs, but not all of them have done so in the same way. Instead of creating a distinctive organizational culture with a more conservative practice style, many of the new plans seek discounts from fee-for-service physicians and use financial incentives to reduce supplier-controlled demand. Financial incentives do affect costs, but whether these organizations are as successful as other HMOs in maintaining and improving the quality of care is less clear.

As a result of legislation passed in 1973, the federal government began providing start-up grants to HMOs and requiring firms with more than twenty-five employees to offer at least one qualified HMO as part of an employee health plan. Congress also revised Medicare to encourage HMO enrollment among the elderly. All of these measures have had a troubled history. The grants program ended in 1981, and Medicare's HMO provisions have failed to bring about any major shift of the elderly into prepaid plans. The requirement that employers offer a qualified HMO is still in effect, but HMOs are reluctant to force employers to comply. Yet while continuing to face enormous difficulties, HMOs have grown in number and enrollment—slowly in the East and the South, more rapidly in the West. This expansion of prepaid plans is probably the single most significant change in the underlying organization of medical care in recent decades.

Managed Care, Unmanaged Competition

The original concept of an alternative health care delivery system—epitomized by the prototype prepaid group practices, such as Kaiser—has been transformed over the past two decades into a broader and looser concept of "managed care." The first step was the inclusion of IPAs under the HMO rubric; then came the addition of the gatekeeper plans. A still looser alternative, preferred provider networks, gives subscribers more complete coverage when they use approved physicians and hospitals that have agreed to accept the plan's rates. While exercising some selective control over providers, provider networks differ from HMOs in that they provide partial out-of-plan coverage for their enrollees. Even fee-for-service insurance plans with utilization review are now described (to my regret) as "managed care." Managed

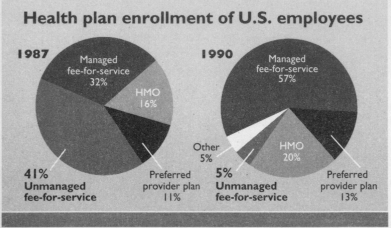

Health plan enrollment of U.S. employees

1987
Managed fee-for-service 32%
HMO 16%
41% Unmanaged fee-for-service
Preferred provider plan 11%

1990
Managed fee-for-service 57%
Other 5%
HMO 20%
5% Unmanaged fee-for-service
Preferred provider plan 13%

SOURCES: *HEALTH AFFAIRS*, WINTER 1991; U.S. CONGRESSIONAL BUDGET OFFICE

Although the percentage of employed Americans covered by all forms of managed care has grown sharply, the largest growth has been in plans that rely on traditional payment arrangements.

care thus no longer refers only to capitation payment plans but also embraces—at least in the emerging conventional usage—any health plan that limits the choice of providers or regulates their treatment decisions to eliminate inappropriate care and reduce costs (see chart).

Given this diversity, it is not possible to generalize about the overall record of managed care. Prepaid group practices—the organizations for which genuine savings and high quality have been most convincingly demonstrated—now represent only a minority of enrollment in managed care plans. Some of the newer plans may achieve savings solely by getting discounts from providers (who may then shift costs elsewhere), by denying approval for care or for payment (at times when, at least according to subscriber complaints, the care may have been needed), and by enrolling healthier people.

The purpose of broadening the concept of prepaid

group practice into managed care was to create a greater variety of health plans, suitable to a great diversity of circumstances and preferences. But in the process, the image of managed care has become confused and perhaps even poisoned. Many patients and doctors now associate the concept of managed care with a form of remote control—a nurse or bureaucrat at the end of a telephone line refusing to approve payment for a service. Many health care executives as well as doctors identify managed care with a form of high-pressure sales organization demanding discounts—personified, as a hospital manager once told me, by the M.B.A. with 10,000 patients in his briefcase who expects, and gets, lower rates.

To be sure, HMOs and other alternatives were bound to create some unhappiness on the part of health care providers, but they were also supposed to generate savings to employers and, ultimately, consumers. Yet the multiple choice arrangements introduced by many companies to allow their employees to choose between one or more managed care plans and conventional insurance have often failed to bring the anticipated savings.

The dynamic at work here was, in fact, quite predictable. Under multiple choice, older and less healthy employees—the ones for whom HMOs might achieve the greatest economies in care—tend to remain in the more traditional, fee-for-service insurance plans. As the costs of these options rise, the managed care plans are able to shadow price (that is, to raise their rates right behind the price leaders), using the additional revenue to provide better benefits as well as higher profits. As a result, the total cost of all plans may be even higher than it would be if the employer offered conventional insurance alone. In addition, many employers still pay the entire premium for all options, effectively removing any cost consciousness from consumer choices.

The problem here is not with the original concept of prepaid health care but with some of the variations on the idea and the inability of employers to counteract the strategies of health plans aimed at escaping responsibility for high-cost patients. It takes hard work for a health plan to produce high-quality care at a lower price; it is much easier to cut costs by attracting healthy subscribers and getting discounts from providers. Unmanaged competition, therefore, generates a lot of cream skimming and discounting, which can be highly profitable for the managed care plan without doing anything to solve the overall problem of health care inflation.

The apparent failure of the competitive approach to contain health costs is, in a sense, not so different from the apparent failure of the regulatory approach. Halfway reform often does not even reach half way. The critics of each approach have been quick to leap upon the initial evidence to pronounce the very principles of regulatory limitation and competitive markets at fault. In the early 1980s, some said regulation had been proven ineffective; ten years later, others said the verdict on competition was the same. But recent experience admits of another interpretation. The regulatory approach failed because it fell short of setting comprehensive budgetary limits, did not control investment, and failed to change incentives. The competitive approach failed because the typical framework established by employers created incentives for opportunism instead of better performance. If we are to get regulatory or competitive strategies right, we have to understand clearly the logic on which they rest.

CHAPTER 4

THE LOGIC OF
SYSTEMIC REFORM

Nothing about health care reform is more fixed in the public mind than the idea that any improvement will be costly. To be sure, reforms that simply add insurance coverage without altering the financing system would cause spending to rise. But that is not necessarily true of structural reforms that provide greater financial control over health care—especially compared with a truly expensive policy: doing nothing.

If we do nothing, national health expenditures are projected to reach $1 trillion in 1994 and to hit $1.65 trillion by the year 2000. Americans, who were spending $2,604 per person on health care in 1990, will be spending $3,920 in 1995 and $5,820 per person in 2000. In 1990 the average worker would have earned about $1,000 more if health care costs had not risen as a share of compensation over the previous fifteen years;

by 2000, at present rates, the average worker will lose another $600 in wages. Thus the cost of any plan must be judged against the backdrop of a system that is running up a larger bill each year without reform.

Although analysts disagree about how much might be saved, international comparisons and detailed studies of health care practices and organizations suggest that the potential economies to be found in the U.S. system— clinical as well as administrative—are enormous. The challenge of health reform is not to persuade the public to give up beneficial care but to reduce the costs that have no benefit, thereby freeing up the resources needed to include the uninsured within a mainstream standard of health coverage.

Ultimately, this means not just changes in health policy but an internal transformation in health care. The true objective of systemic reform is to reach deep inside the process of health care and alter the way all parties concerned—doctors, patients, managers—think about the decisions they face. At the core of the process are the practice styles that shape the everyday choices of physicians about when to order tests, hospitalization, surgery, prescriptions, further visits. Reform works best when it promotes a high-quality but conservative practice style—conservative in the sense of conserving resources by proceeding with treatment only when clearly effective. And it is most likely to succeed when doctors, managers, and other health care professionals work together with patients to arrive at judgments about care through a cooperative rather than antagonistic process.

But how can a more conservative practice style and, I might add, a more conservative style of health care management be achieved? A changed orientation will not spring up naturally, certainly not under the present system, which has richly rewarded the opposite practices.

Nor will it suffice to create public or private regulatory mechanisms that focus on the exceptional cases of gross inefficiency. The crux of the problem is accepted, everyday decision making.

Two approaches offer what I believe to be the best chance of inducing a conservative shift in health care practices and a slowdown in spending. One approach calls for budgetary control from the center, the other for competitive organizations generating decentralized cost sensitivity. Much has been written about each, often exaggerating the contrast between them. In fact, the two approaches have certain similarities; where they differ, they help remedy their respective weaknesses. A coherent strategy for health reform needs to draw on both.

The Logic of Global Caps

To control rising health costs, most major Western countries have eventually found their way to one device: global budgeting, that is, an annually negotiated cap on total expenditures. A global budget may apply to a region, a population, a group of providers, a particular hospital—or, as I shall suggest later, to a private health plan responsible for the comprehensive care of its members. Global budgeting is consistent with a wide variety of ways of organizing health care. It does not necessarily imply a government takeover of health care finance—in the German system negotiations among nongovernmental groups set the caps—but it does require enforceable rules about expenditure limits.

Global budgeting also does not mean centralizing detailed budget decisions; rather, it calls only for setting budget ceilings (thus the word "cap"). Ultimately, such ceilings can result in less government regulation than we have today. Once government, employers, and the public are assured that total health care expenditures will stay within a predetermined limit, they are less likely to pursue the kind of microregulation of health care that the United States has adopted over the past two decades. Global caps, therefore, can be more consistent with both the public interest in controlling costs and the professional interest in maintaining clinical freedom. To borrow a metaphor from two physicians who advocate national health insurance, Kevin Grumbach and Thomas Bodenheimer, microregulation is like tying a leash to every cow in a pasture, while global budgeting is like building a fence. Good fences make leashes unnecessary.

Global caps create a source of countervailing pressure against the health sector's internal impetus toward expansion. The approach seeks to impose a "hard" budget constraint on the providers (or the organizations that pay them), to force them to manage within limits. The intent here is to produce not just fiscal control but new decision making environments, where health care managers and professionals come to accept the need to adopt more conservative practices to match available resources to needs.

Thus the aim is to change not just the economics but also the psychology of health care decisions. The current reimbursement system sets no clear limits; for providers, the object of the reimbursement game is to milk the different sources of payment and, when one resists, to shift costs elsewhere. A comprehensive cap, however, precludes manipulation of the reimbursement system and encourages managers and physicians to concentrate instead on using resources well. Instead of promoting an aggressive therapeutic style and an emphasis on high-cost procedures, global caps encourage less resource-intensive practices that enable providers to manage under constraint. Facing caps, doctors and managers are likely to "internalize" the constraints, gradually altering their rules of thumb about when surgery is really needed or when an expensive new technology genuinely justifies the investment. America's traditional payment system has nurtured therapeutic activism ("when in doubt, take it out"); budget limits nurture therapeutic skepticism ("let's wait and see how this develops"). Given the abundant evidence of excessive surgery, overprescribing, and unnecessary hospitalization, a strong dose of skepticism seems overdue.

Global budgeting for hospitals and for physicians in independent practice has typically involved two different approaches. A global budget for a hospital means a prospectively set, lump-sum payment, instead of reimbursement for itemized services (DRGs are a step in that direction). On the other hand, global budgeting for private physicians, at least on the German model, means annual negotiations between payers and doctors to predetermine a total compensation pool. Physicians bill into the pool under a relative value scale and are paid fee-for-service, with fees being adjusted in midyear corrections to keep overall payments in line with the budget. (This is similar to an IPA.) Doctors who overbill do not threaten the insurance funds or the public treasury; they take money away from their colleagues. Consequently, the government can let the profession decide for itself how it wants to handle such problems.

Global budgeting should be sharply distinguished from price regulation. Price regulation does not guarantee control of total costs because it allows providers to increase the volume of services or shift the mix toward services that are more complex and higher in cost. Nor is a global budget the same as an expenditure target; if the budget constraint is not hard, it is not a real constraint and will not bring about changes in practice patterns.

Global budgeting should also be distinguished from the rationing of medical care, if that is understood as a scheme for limiting beneficial care according to a scale of priorities, as Oregon has proposed for part of its Medicaid program. The Oregon approach would rank procedures according to likely benefit, cutting off payment for those below a line dictated by available funds. Because of the crude nature of the Oregon ranking—for example, it fails to take the patient's prognosis into account—the system would sometimes deny care to patients with a chance of recovery and approve it for others who have none. By regulating specific clinical situations, Oregon's plan calls for a highly intrusive level of state control. Global budgeting may require tough choices, but it leaves such decisions outside the state to the changing judgments and negotiations of health plan managers, doctors, and patients (although it can and should provide for an appeals process, based on public and professional standards). This approach avoids the rigidity of detailed official rules that are likely to become outdated as new scientific discoveries emerge.

Critics of global budgeting often liken it to "command and control" central planning. But on closer inspection, it involves a great deal of decentralization. It is true, however, that as global budgeting is usually carried out, it involves regulation of capital investment and planning of health facilities, to prevent duplication and keep the long-range growth of expenditures in check. In some regions, this may be the best approach. Since the demand for health care depends on the available supply, much of the focus of cost control must take the form of "managed capacity"—that is, gearing the resources of a region or health plan to the needs of the population. The disadvantage of publicly determined investment controls is that they may block competition and lock patterns of health care in place; and when the planning forecasts are wrong, shortages may be the result.

There are two other serious objections to global budgeting. On its own, global budgeting does not ensure that cost control is achieved through improved efficiency rather than reduced services and lengthened waiting lines. Improved efficiency depends on building into the system rewards for better performance and penalties for worse.

Perhaps more serious, the costs of health care in the United States are already on a sharp upward trajectory, partly because of policies that have expanded physician training, hospital construction, and medical research. Seventy percent of American doctors are specialists; countries with successful global budgeting typically have half their doctors in primary care. While we may try to impose a global budget, the powerful expansionary pressures already at work in the American health care system may just bust the lid off. That prospect suggests we need some other force, working from below, generating other changes to make the system more efficient, innovative, and responsive to consumer choice.

The Logic of Managed Competition
Managed competition, the design for reform introduced in 1977 by Alain Enthoven, is one of several models for using market forces to control health costs and improve the system's performance. The basic idea is to get groups of providers to compete with each other in a framework that allows consumers to choose intelligently among them and that encourages cost-conscious decision making. Unlike some other market approaches, the success of managed competition does not

depend on the implausible possibility that consumers
will shop around for care when they are sick, nor does
it call for higher deductibles and copayments as a way
of creating greater patient sensitivity to costs. Rather,
the key decision point is the annual choice of a health
plan, a choice made at a time when consumers are not
under pressures of illness and can evaluate alternative
plans at different prices. Under managed competition,
these alternatives would consist of HMOs and other
managed care plans, as well as a conventional insurance plan offering choice of any willing provider as
long as that option is able to survive in a competitive
framework.

For consumers to make informed choices among
these alternatives, the choices need to be presented
clearly, with prices that reflect true differences in the
plans, not in their enrollees. This is the job of the
"sponsor." (Under the current system, the sponsor is
typically an employer, although in some cases it is a
government agency.) The sponsor negotiates the benefits
packages, conducts the annual enrollment, provides information to consumers, and collects and disburses payments to plans. Ideally, the sponsor is not merely
passive but instead "manages" the competition—hence
the name.

Health plan competition has to be managed because it
is susceptible to several predictable problems. Health
plans can reduce their costs most easily by avoiding
high-risk subscribers; thus they have an incentive to discriminate against the chronically ill and disabled and
any group believed to be high-risk. To gain a more favorable "risk selection," the plans may even refuse to
provide benefits or special services that attract such
high-cost groups as alcoholics, HIV-infected individuals,
and the mentally ill. Thus without regulation, a compet-

itive market may well drive out services for the very people who need health care the most. Furthermore, consumers may have difficulty making informed choices among health plans if there are complex variations in benefits, cost-sharing, exclusions, and so on.

The ground rules of managed competition are designed to overcome these problems.

First, there must be *open enrollment* by consumers. Health plans that want to offer coverage must offer it to everyone; they cannot just take the healthy and affluent. Nor can they arbitrarily drop subscribers or deny coverage for preexisting conditions. And to prevent plans from marketing to the healthy and avoiding the sick, the sponsor must conduct the enrollment process independent of any plan.

Second, the approach calls for creating a *standard, comprehensive benefits package* to prevent health plans from shaping their benefits packages to attract low-risk subscribers and to enable consumers to make easy price comparisons. (This does not prevent plans from offering supplementary packages, although these must be priced to reflect their full cost.)

Third, the competing health plans must agree to be *accountable for the quality of the care* they provide. That means regular monitoring of both the objective outcomes of care and consumer satisfaction and publication of the results.

Fourth, the approach calls for *cost-conscious choice*. Consumers should reap the savings from any plan that can produce the standard benefits at a lower cost, and they should be asked to pay the marginal difference of any plan that produces those benefits at a higher cost. Thus employers and government should make a fixed-dollar contribution that does not vary according to the plan a consumer selects. Consumers would pay the difference between that contribution and the premium of their chosen plan.

Fifth, the approach calls for *community rating* premiums for consumers and *risk-adjusting* payments to plans. The same community-wide rates would apply to all consumers; premiums would not be higher for those who are older or for people with disabilities or preexisting conditions. However, the sponsors would pay the plans according to the risk of the populations they enroll. They would make an upward adjustment in payments to plans attracting older or sicker subscribers and adjust downward payments to plans enrolling lower-risk subscribers. The purpose of this measure is to reduce the incentive to skim off the healthiest and avoid the sick. In addition, the sponsor would have discretionary authority to counteract any opportunistic behavior by plans that attempt to skim off the healthy or disenroll consumers with high-cost illnesses.

These policies are crucial both to control costs and to avoid the inequity—and irrationality—of a health insurance system, such as ours today, that avoids sick people. One reason for the failure of current multiple choice plans set up by employers, as I suggested earlier, is that they have not been able to structure the competition appropriately. When the prices of alternative plans reflect the risk of the people who enroll, the price system does not send the right signals. Instead of attracting consumers to the most efficient providers, competition currently attracts consumers to the healthiest risk pools. The winning plan may well be inefficient in providing health care but clever at marketing.

Thus while managed competition draws on the strengths of a market system, it also must guard against its potential failures. Managed competition requires carefully structured rules, plus a sufficient concentration

Global caps vs. managed competition

WHAT THEY HAVE IN COMMON
- Create expenditure limits
- Encourage conservative practice styles
- Reduce microregulation of providers
- Use countervailing power to control costs

WHERE THEY DIFFER

GLOBAL BUDGET CAPS	MANAGED COMPETITION
Extensive experience in other countries	Distinctively American
Reliance on planning for efficiency and innovation	Market-based incentives for efficiency and innovation
Feasible in every region	Not feasible everywhere

of people in a region to support competing health plans. Competition is not a magic bullet that dispenses with health care regulation.

Like global budgeting, managed competition moves health care into a world of expenditure limits. Indeed, capitation payment produces a more global budget than do the Canadian and German health insurance systems, since a health plan paid by capitation works under a comprehensive budget constraint, not just a budget cap on hospital care or physicians' services separately. This is actually a source of greater flexibility: Capitation enables health plans to reallocate resources from inpatient to ambulatory services in line with changing preferences and new technology and to introduce nontraditional providers, such as nurse practitioners, in lieu of physicians.

Like global budgeting, managed competition generates greater countervailing power to offset provider-induced demand. It also promotes a framework of decision making in which managers, physicians, and other providers have incentives to use more conservative practices. In this model, the impetus comes not only from a hard budget constraint, but also from the threat of competition, which pushes the HMOs and other managed care plans to match their resources to the needs of their enrolled membership.

The merits of managed competition depend on the kinds of health plans that would grow under the system. As I have suggested, HMOs today include many of the best health care organizations in the country. They have shown that it is indeed possible to provide high-quality care at significantly lower cost. But not all managed care plans today exhibit those virtues, and unfortunately, the dominant HMOs in some areas are not admirable organizations. When based on multispecialty group practices, HMOs are most likely to pursue lower costs and higher quality through the cooperative involvement of their physicians in developing conservative practice patterns. But when based on doctors in independent, fee-for-service practice, the health plans are much more likely to keep costs under control by pressuring doctors to discount their fees and by requiring telephone approval of hospitalization and other procedures. The result is more likely to be an adversarial relationship, in which physicians—and their patients—feel they are subject to control by a remote bureaucracy.

Thus the success of managed competition in a region will be greatly affected by its patterns of medical practice and the capacity of health care institutions to move from adversarial to cooperative forms of organization. At present, managed competition seems more likely to work in the cities and suburbs of the West, where group practice is more common, than in the older metropolitan areas of the East, where solo, fee-for-service practice still prevails. Throughout the country, managed competition also faces limits in rural areas, where it is often difficult to get a single health care provider, much less competing alternatives. As a result, managed competition is not an approach that can instantly—or ever—be used everywhere.

Combining the Approaches

Most analysts of health policy take the two approaches I have been describing to lead in two opposite directions: global budgeting, toward a single-payer system of national health insurance; managed competition, toward a private sector model. But to pose such a stark choice is misleading.

Any single-payer plan in the United States would have to provide for capitation payment to HMOs and other managed care plans. If there is capitation, there is the prospect of competition. Competition raises the problem of risk selection and the need to counteract any opportunistic tendency of plans to skim off the healthy and avoid the sick. Consequently, even single-payer plans would have to figure out how to manage health plan competition.

On the other hand, managed competition does not preclude expenditure limits. As I have suggested, capitation payment is a kind of global budgeting. Consequently, it is entirely possible to have both budget limitation and competition. The California Public Employee Retirement System (CalPERS), covering 900,000 people, has been one of the leading prototypes of a budgeted system that promotes competition among private health plans. The Federal Employees Health Benefit Program also has some of the same elements. A universal health plan that promotes competition under a budget can do as well—indeed, it can do even better.

Thus despite sharp ideological differences among their advocates, the single-payer model of national health insurance and managed competition are not wholly opposed. To be sure, the single-payer model treats competing HMOs as an incidental feature (and may provide little incentive to use them), whereas the pro-competitive model seeks to assure quality and control of costs by forcing plans to compete by price and service. But even the most ardent advocates of managed competition must recognize that there are geographic and other barriers to carrying out the idea throughout the country. Where managed competition is impractical, or where the infrastructure of competitive health plans has yet to develop, global budgeting by a single payer may be the best—albeit second best—method of containing costs.

The United States faces fundamentally different circumstances today compared to other countries at the time they developed universal coverage. Costs are dramatically higher; the organization of health care has changed. When Canada and the European countries developed their national health insurance programs, they generally accepted the existing method of fee-for-service payment for physicians. Had the U.S. adopted national health insurance decades ago, it too would have premised its system on fee-for-service medicine. But with the rise of HMOs and managed care plans, the U.S. has now developed a different structure. It would be a mistake, as well as hopeless, to try to turn back the clock, because a system based on capitation payment and organized systems of care has important advantages.

But the establishment of global budgeting and managed competition and the achievement of universal coverage face a major obstacle: the existing framework of employment-based insurance. If systemic reform is to mean anything, it must mean transforming that system.

CHAPTER 5

BREAKING THE
JOB LINKAGE

Most Americans get health coverage through a job—their own or that of some member of their family. Employment is the port of entry, therefore, not only for most consumers but also for health care reform. Under the current system, employers not only pay a share of insurance premiums; they also determine the kinds of health plans offered to most Americans and the framework of choice among plans and providers. But in today's health insurance market, this raises serious questions: Should Americans' access to health care, and the price they pay for it, depend on the vagaries of the job market, the size of their firm, and their employer's benefit policies? Should employers be burdened with managing their employees' health care? Are employers the best agents for making these decisions?

Employers began offering health insurance as a fringe

benefit half a century ago, scarcely imagining how much cloth that fringe might ultimately take. The employment-based system has persisted since then, due less to positive belief than to inertia and the difficulty of gaining consensus on an alternative. Today few on the right or the left defend the employers' role in the provision of health insurance as a matter of principle. "If we were beginning with a blank slate," many in health policy say, "we would not have an employer-based system. But it's not practical to change it."

This argument is losing force as well as conviction. Employers today do not derive any great benefit from mediating the purchase of health insurance. Many would dearly love to be rid of the burden. Managed care, moreover, involves employers in regulating their employees' personal choices and creates new sources of tension and resentment. As those problems grow, many firms are likely to begin asking why they ever became involved in choosing doctors and hospitals for their workers and families when they do not choose their schools or housing or make other personal choices for them.

The Costs of the Job Linkage

Employment-based health insurance has always had drawbacks, although some have become apparent only with time.

First, and most obviously, gaining access to health insurance depends on whether a member of the household is employed and what kind of employment that person has. Part-time and seasonal jobs generally do not qualify for benefits. Children and spouses of employees receive insurance only indirectly, incidentally, and haphazardly. In recent years, the limitations of employment-based coverage of children have become especially severe. Between 1977 and 1992 the proportion of children covered by employer-based coverage dropped from 72.8 percent to 60.2 percent. Employer-based insurance thus fails to cover nearly 26 million children—four of every ten.

Second, the employee group now forms the key risk pool for determining health insurance premiums. Partly because of demographic differences among these groups, some people receive relatively low insurance rates, while others face rates that are prohibitively high. Among the losers are those who work for small firms, for firms with relatively older workers, and in occupations believed to create high health risks or to attract workers from high-risk groups. Not surprisingly, the largest decline in employment-based coverage has recently been among workers in small firms. Between 1991 and 1992, 42 percent of the additional 2.2 million uninsured Americans belonged to families headed by people employed by firms with fewer than twenty-five workers.

Third, the system gives employers decision making power over insurance and medical care. Under traditional insurance plans—those that allow the insured free choice of provider and impose few controls—the employer's power is a relatively minor concern. But the rise of health costs has led many employers into micromanaging the health care of their employees' families or selecting agents to do so. This change raises concerns about infringements on liberty and privacy.

Fourth, the tax subsidy of employer-provided insurance is much greater for higher-income than for lower-income Americans. For a family in the 15 percent tax bracket, the exclusion from taxable income of a dollar in employer-paid health benefits is worth only 15 cents. For a family in the 40 percent tax bracket, the same exclusion is worth 40 cents. The subsidy also goes dispro-

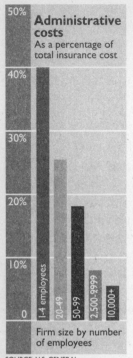

Administrative costs
As a percentage of total insurance cost

50%
40%
30%
20%
10%
0

1-4 employees
20-49
50-99
2,500-9,999
10,000+

Firm size by number of employees

SOURCE: U.S. GENERAL ACCOUNTING OFFICE

Smaller companies may pay as much as 40 percent of insurance premiums for administration, as opposed to actual health services. Large companies may pay less than 10 percent.

portionately to the affluent because the higher their income, the more likely Americans are to get insurance from their employer and the more generous those benefits tend to be. In 1991, according to an estimate by Lewin-VHI, the average value of the tax break to a family with a $100,000 income was $1,500, while the benefit to families with incomes below $10,000 averaged $50. Thus people with the best private insurance coverage get the most federal help to pay for it.

Fifth, employers have shown little ability to control health costs over the long run. Periodically, during cycles in the insurance market, costs have slowed down and observers have declared victory over health care inflation—only to see costs shoot up a few years later. The chief effect of employers' cost-containment efforts has been not to reduce costs but to shift them back to their employees and sometimes to other individuals with private insurance who have less clout in the marketplace.

Sixth, the employer-based insurance system generates extraordinarily high administrative costs. While Medicare's administrative costs run about 3 percent, private insurers absorb about 13 cents of every premium dollar in marketing and other administrative costs, taxes, and profits—a figure that does not include the administrative costs to the employer, much less to employees and their families. The share of insurance premiums consumed by administration is especially high for medium-size and small employers. For firms with fewer than fifty workers, insurance companies absorb about 25 cents of every premium dollar; for firms with five or fewer workers, insurers take 40 cents (see chart, opposite page).

Seventh, employer-provided insurance has adverse effects on labor-management relations and employment. The system entangles employers in conflicts over health care, drains management time, and leads employers to make increasing use of uninsured part-time and contract workers, who enjoy few rights and little security.

Some may disagree with one or another of the foregoing points. But many conservatives as well as liberals agree that access to insurance ought not to depend on the particular firm one works for, that the tax subsidy is inequitable, and that it is doubtful whether individual employers can control costs. The first question of reform, therefore, is whether it is possible to adjust public policies to remedy the many deficiencies of the employment-based system. To answer that question, it helps to understand why employment-based insurance developed in the first place.

Why We Have an Employment-Based System

The linkage of health insurance to employment originally helped to launch and then to broaden insurance protection against the costs of sickness. Until the 1930s, insurance companies did not offer health coverage because the losses appeared impossible to predict. The insurers feared *adverse selection* (people with high expected costs would be the most likely to take out policies). They foresaw high marketing expenses and collection problems (collecting life insurance payments at the time typically required door-to-door agents). And they were concerned about the risk that health insurance would not just spread costs but increase them, because the insured would seek more medical care and doctors would raise fees.

This last problem, known as "moral hazard," was never really solved. But the sale of health insurance to employee groups rather than individuals—pioneered by Blue Cross plans, which hospital associations launched during the Depression—did make private health insurance a workable proposition. Because the employed are a relatively healthy population, group insurance limited adverse selection; the introduction of automatic payroll deductions guaranteed payment of premiums and cut marketing and collection costs. By the late 1930s, commercial insurers had entered the market.

When national health insurance plans failed to pass Congress during the New Deal and the Truman years, employment-based health insurance took off, encouraged by World War II-era wage-price controls that exempted employer-paid health insurance premiums and by federal tax policies that excluded the employer's health insurance contributions from taxable income. Unions demanded health insurance in collective bargaining, and employers agreed to provide it to attract and keep good workers.

Employment-related insurance grew steadily through the postwar period until the late 1970s. Then the percentage of employed Americans who lack health insurance began to increase. Partly because employment has shifted from manufacturing to services and unions have declined, jobs with health benefits have been stagnant, while jobs without benefits have grown. The rollback of health insurance, like the decline of pension coverage, reflects the now indisputable shrinkage of middle-class jobs in the U.S.

The dynamics of the insurance market have also been

a factor in declining health coverage. From their beginnings in the 1930s, Blue Cross plans offered health insurance to all employers in a geographic area at the same price, a method known as community rating. Commercial insurance companies, however, provided lower rates to healthier employee groups on the basis of their cost experience (hence the term "experience rating"). This threatened to leave the Blues with the highest-cost subscribers and forced the plans to move away from community rating. In recent decades, insurers have discriminated ever more carefully among groups bearing different risks. This practice, known as market segmentation, inevitably results in the exclusion from coverage of those judged especially high-risk. Today's private insurance system is the outcome of this evolution.

Can this patient—employer-sponsored insurance—be saved? That's what a variety of proposals attempt to do. *Insurance market reform* would change laws regarding rating practices and other features of the existing private market. *Voluntary public insurance* or *publicly subsidized private insurance*, often via *tax credits*, would either supplement current coverage with a public program or subsidize the purchase of private insurance in the current system. Some recent proposals also include an *individual mandate* that would require every individual to purchase some minimum level of coverage. *Mandated employer benefits* would require employers to cover their workers or, as in play-or-pay proposals, to choose between providing coverage or paying into a public program. Proposals for incremental (as opposed to systemic) reform often combine several of these components in the effort to achieve universal coverage while preserving the role of employers as decision makers about health insurance.

The Limits of Insurance Market Reform

The purpose of reforming the insurance market is to reverse its recent evolution, recreating a wider distribution of risk. The leading proposals—some of which have been adopted in New York and other states—would prohibit the use of preexisting condition exclusions at least in group policies, require the renewal of policies without regard to new illnesses, and either require community rating or limit the range of experience rating to reduce prices to groups judged high-risk. Some proposals would also limit annual premium increases.

The political appeal of these measures is clear. They do not require new taxes to cover the uninsured; instead, they force the insurance industry to reduce prices to high-risk groups and to insure some people now denied coverage. Yet there are some obvious problems.

First, forcing insurers to community rate and accept all applicants means that while rates will go down for some small firms and high-risk individuals, they will go up for the majority of people who are now insured (unless other measures simultaneously control costs). Once rate increases hit these people, they may conclude that the government has bungled things again.

Second, proposals for community rating usually continue to allow employers to self-insure; thus the "community" that receives the same insurance rates consists of the residual population, which typically has higher costs.

Third, while government can regulate insurance rates, it is difficult to force private insurance companies to cover high-risk groups they prefer to avoid. Instead, they may adopt ever more subtle risk-avoidance strategies, making it difficult for many people to get insurance. States that create community-rated pools for

individuals and small groups that otherwise cannot purchase insurance may find the rates offered by insurers
are prohibitively high. If they try to put all insurance
into such pools, more companies will self-insure to escape the pools and insurers may threaten to withdraw
from the states' health insurance business altogether.

Even comprehensive insurance market reform would
still leave millions uninsured. Moreover, it would do
nothing to control overall health care costs or to reduce
administrative waste. At most it would help employees
of some small businesses and people with preexisting
conditions to get coverage at more affordable rates and
to avoid job lock. However, any attempt to impose community rates without requiring universal coverage and a
broad, communitywide pooling of risk will guarantee
that insurers demand high premiums to compensate for
adverse selection. And if health costs continue to soar,
those who benefit from these reforms in the short run
will merely face the same problems of unaffordable rates
a bit later.

Subsidies without Employer Mandates
Yet another approach is to extend insurance through direct public subsidies for coverage of the uninsured without mandating any employer participation. There are
several options here. The government can:

- subsidize private insurers to provide coverage of
  high-risk individuals;
- allow the uninsured to buy subsidized coverage
  from Medicaid;
- set up an entirely separate public insurance plan to
  provide affordable policies to people otherwise uninsured; or
- provide tax credits to the poor to buy insurance.

The immediate difficulty with all such approaches is their cost. Without employer contributions, the government must raise other taxes to secure the revenue required to cover the working poor. Moreover, if employees can get coverage at reasonable rates from a public program without an employer contribution, employers will have an incentive to drop health benefits. As a result, the costs of a public program are likely to grow, perhaps to unmanageable proportions. Such a program would also have high costs because it would cover many people deemed uninsurable by private companies. The combined effect of covering high-risk individuals denied private insurance and inducing employers to drop benefits tends to make such approaches fiscally unsustainable. In addition, many people eligible for public insurance would still decline to pay for it, even at subsidized rates, preferring to take their chances and to use public hospitals if they need care. The result would likely be severe adverse selection: Those who purchase coverage will be disproportionately people with high expected costs.

Nonetheless, many states are experimenting with such approaches. About half the states have created subsidized high-risk insurance pools; several others, such as Maine, are subsidizing coverage of the uninsured directly. Typically, these programs do not reach all of the uninsured; in most cases they reach only a small minority at costs so high that there is no likelihood that they will be extended to cover all the uninsured. Minnesota is one state that has attempted to cover most of the uninsured this way, but it has a big advantage: The percentage of Minnesotans without insurance is much lower than the national average. Hence the scale of the problem is smaller; even so, the Minnesota program, which involves a new state insurance program, will not reach everyone and may cause smaller employers to dump their health benefits obligations on the taxpayers.

An individual mandate would reduce the problem of adverse selection, but it would create formidable problems of its own. Without any employer contribution, many families would face a staggering burden; subsidies would have to reach roughly half the population (with attendant administrative problems). Employers would then cut back coverage, generating still higher subsidy costs. Thus while attempting to leave the existing employer-based system in place, this approach risks destabilizing it.

To minimize the cost of subsidies, the mandated coverage could be kept to a barebones or catastrophic level, but this has its own problems. It discourages use of preventive and primary care and blocks a shift in the delivery system toward greater emphasis on those services. Catastrophic insurance reinforces the skewed allocation of resources toward high-cost services that has made the American health system the most costly in the world.

Mandates without Change
One way to extend health coverage is to require all employers to offer it. Absent more comprehensive reforms, however, employer mandates do not solve the problems of rising costs and pose serious problems for small and medium-size businesses. For while large employers pay as little as 6 percent of payroll for health insurance, smaller firms pay as much as 12 or 14 percent, or even more.

Hawaii is the one state that requires all employers to offer health insurance. In 1975, shortly after the enactment of the federal Employment Security and Retirement Act (ERISA), which regulates employee benefit plans, Hawaii adopted its health insurance mandate. Several years later, after a federal court held the mandate in violation of ERISA, Hawaii's representatives persuaded

Congress to give the state a special exemption to maintain its system. By most accounts, it has been a success: Hawaii not only has close to universal health insurance, but health care costs are below the national average. In some respects, Hawaii seems to be a special case because of its isolation from the mainland and the dominant role in its health care played by two large competing plans. But the ability of its small employers to pass on the costs of health insurance suggests that small business fears of mandated benefits are exaggerated.

Nonetheless, to quiet those fears and to reduce the potential for adverse business and employment effects, proposals for mandatory benefits have generally come in combination with other measures, such as insurance market reform (to cut down private insurance rates quoted to small firms) or an option for employers to buy public insurance at an affordable price. Under the latter play-or-pay approach, the controlled price of the public program would effectively put a cap on the employer's obligations.

Twenty years ago, when health costs were much lower, public coverage for uninsured working Americans might have cost as little as 4 percent of payroll. (That was the tax rate in national health insurance proposals of the mid-1970s.) Today a payroll tax at that level would not come close to covering employees and their families, much less the unemployed and those outside the labor force. The play-or-pay legislation proposed in 1990 by leading Democrats included a formula for determining the price to the employer of public coverage that would have set the rate at between 8 and 9 percent of payroll. At that level, there would likely have been a large public program, enrolling between a third and a half of the population under age sixty-five. Others would have been covered by insurance purchased directly by employers.

The difficulties with this approach are fundamental. It

would tend to divide Americans into two classes, with the lower tier in the public program likely to have fewer benefits and lower standards. The structure of play-or-pay, moreover, gives employers, not employees, the power to decide which option to take. Hence many Americans would fear their employer "dumping" them into a public program akin to Medicaid. In other words, while play-or-pay would be a step up for the millions who have no insurance, it would appear to be a step down for the millions who do.

Of course, the public program would not have to be like Medicaid. But it would be likely to attract higher-risk individuals and relatively higher-cost groups, raising its costs relative to private insurance. In addition, the class makeup of the participants in the public program would suggest it was the less desirable option. Voters with employer-provided insurance would have an interest only in containing the costs of the public program, not in improving it; hence political pressure seems likely to be biased in a restrictive direction.

Beyond Incremental Reform

All the foregoing proposals attempt to build on the foundation of employer-sponsored insurance. This is the strategy of incremental reform. But it is one thing to build on a solid foundation, another to build on a collapsing one. Employment-based insurance is unraveling. And the more employers do try to control health costs, the more they intrude into what ought to be their employees' private decisions about health care.

Even if employer-sponsored managed care were to control costs, it would do nothing to remedy many of the inherent problems of a job-based system. If access to a health plan is tied to a job, the families of employees changing jobs in the same community will often be

Percentage of Workers in Firms with Employer-Sponsored Health Coverage Who Have a Choice of More Than One Type of Plan

1–24 Workers	12%
25–49 Workers	21%
50–99 Workers	24%
100–199 Workers	25%
200–499 Workers	45%
500–999 Workers	63%
1,000–4,999 Workers	67%
5,000+ Workers	99%

SOURCE: KPMG PEAT MARWICK

The majority of employees of small businesses that insure do not have the opportunity to choose among alternative health plans. And many of those who do have a choice can choose only among plans offered by a single insurance company.

forced, as they are today, to change health care plans and providers regardless of whether they are satisfied. Firms will continue to have incentives to discriminate against prospective employees that have family members with disabilities and chronic illnesses. Administrative inefficiencies will not be significantly reduced. Most small and midsize employers do not at present offer their employees a choice of plan (see chart, above), and to require each employer to make multiple arrangements separately would add administrative burdens.

As emphasized earlier, employers also are unlikely to be able to manage competition appropriately. Older employees tend to stick with fee-for-service. As a result, the costs of fee-for-service plans may escalate because of

risk selection. If employers are the sponsors of competition but do not perform any risk adjustment to their
premium payments, the plans providing choice of any
willing provider will likely disappear entirely.

While it is possible in theory to universalize employment-based insurance by providing either tax credits to
individuals or a supplementary public insurance program, these options tend to be extremely costly. They
channel more money into a system that shows no ability
to control its appetite. Paradoxically, it requires public
action to create a workable market in health care.

We need to distinguish, therefore, between the employer's role in *paying* for coverage and the employer's
role in *providing* it. A plausible route to a universal
system cannot avoid maintaining joint employer and
employee contributions for health insurance. That is
the way Americans have come to pay for health insurance; other alternatives represent too great a financial upheaval. However, health coverage may be partly
employer-paid without being job-dependent and employer-provided. National health care reform should aim
at breaking the job linkage that makes access to affordable coverage depend on a job and that puts individual
employers between Americans and their doctors.

Compared with incremental reform of employment-
based insurance, national health insurance—that is, a
system that makes insurance coverage available on the
basis of citizenship rather than employment—would provide greater security, freedom, and economy. Universal
coverage, however, does not mean that the government
has to run the health care system, or that there cannot be
multiple health plans, or that consumers cannot have
choice. That depends on the design of reform.

CHAPTER 6

A NEW FRAMEWORK

The previous two chapters have suggested the outlines of an approach to universal coverage that breaks the linkage of health insurance to jobs and enables consumers to choose among private health plans competing under a budget cap. The most comprehensive program embodying that approach is the plan presented by President Clinton in the fall of 1993.

Like universal health insurance in other countries, the Clinton Health Security plan makes coverage a right of citizenship rather than a fringe benefit of employment. It protects Americans from losing their health coverage if their business fails, they lose their job, they get sick, or their life circumstances change because of divorce, the death of a spouse, or a move to another state. The plan guarantees all citizens and legal residents a comprehensive package of health benefits, prohibits the abusive practices and exclusions that make much insurance today inadequate and unreliable, and sets limits on how rapidly average premiums in a region are allowed to increase.

Unlike the systems of most other countries, however, the Health Security program offers consumers the opportunity to choose among alternative health plans and requires those plans to compete for their enrollment on quality and price. The key institutional innovation expanding choice and restructuring competition is the development of regional health alliances (called "health insurance purchasing cooperatives" in other proposals). Health alliances are not insurers, much less providers of health care. They are purchasers—sponsors—of coverage, responsible for organizing the market and making available to consumers an array of private health plans, each providing a comprehensive benefits package. Except for employees in the very largest companies (those with more than 5,000 employees), the regional purchasing alliances replace employers as the gateways to health insurance, offering most people more alternatives than they now have. Some media reports have said the alliances would offer three plans. In fact, plans offered through the alliances would come in three *types*: traditional fee-for-service insurance, HMOs, and preferred provider networks. There is no limit on the number of plans.

Based on regular monitoring of the outcomes of care and surveys of consumer satisfaction, an annual report card would provide comparative information on each plan's quality and service as well as price. Consumers would choose a plan during the annual open enrollment run by the alliance. Unless a health plan faced capacity limits because of limited facilities or staff, it would have to take all who signed up; under no circumstances would plans be permitted to screen out the sick.

The alliances would receive funds from employers and

Estimated Average Premiums

Policy type		Two-parent family with children	Single-parent family	Couple	Single
Total premium	monthly	$363	$324	$322	$161
	annual	$4,360	$3,893	$3,865	$1,932
Family share*	monthly	$73	$65	$64	$32
	annual	$872	$779	$773	$386

SOURCE: OFFICE OF THE ACTUARY, HEALTH CARE FINANCE ADMINISTRATION

*"Family share" refers to the 20 percent of average premiums owed by individuals or families that receive the minimum employer contribution and no low-income discount.

Preliminary projections for 1994 premiums under the Clinton plan show an average of $4,360 for two-parent families and $1,932 for single individuals.

employees, from others according to their ability to pay, and from government. The funds would flow out to the health plans according to their enrolled population. Employer contributions would pay for a share of the average premium; at a minimum, the employer share would cover 80 percent of the average, though an employer could choose to pay part of the employee share.

Employees would pay the difference between their employer contribution and the premium of their chosen plan. Premiums would vary only according to family status (see chart, above, for projected 1994 average premiums). No consumer would pay more because of any personal characteristic or medical condition. An individual or family that enrolled in an average-cost plan, did not qualify for a low-income discount, and received the minimum 80 percent employer contribution would pay the remaining 20 percent of the premium. For two-parent families, the average premium for 1994 would be $73 a month; for individuals, $32 monthly.

Consumers could, however, pay less by choosing a plan that cost less, and they would pay the extra amount if they preferred a plan that provided the guaranteed benefits package at a higher premium. Consider a hypothetical alliance with five health plans and an average individual premium of $150 a month (see chart, next page). The employer share would be $120; on average, an employee receiving the minimum contribution and no low-income discount would pay $30. However, in this alliance, the employee could pay as little as $15 or as much as $45, depending on which plan he or she chose. The plans would all offer the same scope of services and coverage, but they would vary in their mode of organization, choice of providers, quality of service, and other features. Consumers would have to decide whether a more expensive plan was worth the extra cost.

Because consumers reap the savings when premiums are lower, health plans have an incentive to provide the most value at the lowest premium if they want to build up or even retain their enrollment. Where employees have had incentives to make cost-conscious choices because they pay the marginal cost of a plan—for example, at Xerox, Digital, GTE, and the Minnesota public employee system—many employees have switched out of high-cost plans, and overall costs have fallen.

The Health Security plan also includes several key features that help make coverage affordable to employers. First, by spreading the costs of families, the plan avoids requiring *individual* employers to pay 80 percent of the premium for a family. Because many families include more than one worker, alliances would collect too much money if they asked all employers for 80 percent of the premium for each worker with a family. So, to meet the

Hypothetical Alliance	Monthly Premiums (Individual Policy)		
	Total	Employer*	Employee
Plan 1	$135	$120	$15
Plan 2	$145	$120	$25
Plan 3 (average cost)	$150	$120	$30
Plan 4	$155	$120	$35
Plan 5	$165	$120	$45

* Refers to credit given to a full-time employee for employer contributions, regardless of whether the employer or employers paid that amount. (Some employers' contributions are capped; also, employees are not held liable for employer delinquencies.)

In this hypothetical alliance, an individual employee receiving the minimum employer contribution and no discount for low income may pay from $15 to $45 a month, depending on the plan chosen.

required share, individual employers would pay 80 percent of the family premium *divided by the average number of workers per family in a region*. Nationally, families average 1.4 workers; consequently, the average contribution required of employers would be only 57 percent of the family premium (80 percent divided by 1.4)—or an estimated $2,479 for a family (see chart, next page).

Second, firms participating in the regional alliances—all those with fewer than 5,000 workers—would pay no more than 7.9 percent of payroll for the required employer share. Businesses with fewer than 75 workers would receive discounts reducing their costs to between 3.5 percent and 7.9 percent of payroll, depending on their size and average wages (see chart, next page). The self-employed would be treated as a small business and enjoy the same discounts; they would also be able to deduct 100 percent of their health insurance costs from taxable income.

Low-income households, the unemployed, and early

Estimated Employer Contributions for 1994

Policy type	Two-parent family	Single-parent family	Couple	Single
EMPLOYER SHARE	$2,479	$2,479	$2,125	$1,546

Caps on Required Employer Contributions as a Percent of Payroll

Average Wage	Size of Firm			
	Under 25 employees	25–49 employees	50–74 employees	75–5,000 employees
Under $12,000	3.5%	4.4%	5.3%	7.9%
$12,000–14,999	4.4%	5.3%	6.2%	7.9%
$15,000–17,999	5.3%	6.2%	7.1%	7.9%
$18,000–20,999	6.2%	7.1%	7.9%	7.9%
$21,000–23,999	7.1%	7.9%	7.9%	7.9%
$24,000–or more	7.9%	7.9%	7.9%	7.9%

SOURCE: CLINTON ADMINISTRATION

The average required employer contribution for a worker with a family would be $2,479 in 1994. For all its workers combined, no firm in the regional alliances would pay more than 7.9 percent of payroll. Small firms are capped at lower levels depending on size and average wages.

retirees would also receive discounts to enable them to choose a plan through the alliances at an affordable rate. Medicaid will cease to provide separate coverage for the poor; its funds will pay for welfare beneficiaries and the disabled who receive Supplemental Security Income (SSI) to enroll in any plan in their regional alliance with a premium up to the average. Others previously covered by Medicaid, such as the "medically needy" who have exhausted their assets paying for medical care, will have been covered under an alliance plan to begin with.

Medicare would remain a separate program, although at age sixty-five retirees could opt to remain in the alliances and pay the difference between the amount Medicare would pay to the plan and its premium for the elderly. The Clinton plan would expand Medicare to include the same coverage of prescription drugs available to the under–sixty-five population.

The Health Security Act also includes support for home- and community-based long-term care for the disabled of all ages, and it calls for new tax incentives and tighter standards for private long-term care insurance. While veterans would retain existing rights to health services run by the Department of Veterans Affairs, the VA would begin transforming its facilities into integrated health plans that could enroll veterans for comprehensive coverage through the alliances. The Department of Defense health care system would also move in the same direction. Coverage of all federal employees would shift to the health alliances; thus members of Congress would get their coverage through the same alliances and health plans as average citizens.

The transition to a reformed system would take place in stages. The Clinton plan phases in universal coverage, state by state, between 1996 and 1998, and defers some elements of the benefits package, notably broader mental health and adult dental coverage, until 2001. Regional caps on premium increases would not go into effect until 1996. The proposed support for home-based long-term care would be introduced gradually between 1996 and 2000.

While establishing a federal framework for financing, coverage, benefits, and consumer protections, the Health Security plan gives the states authority to set up the regional alliances and to adopt a variety of different approaches to controlling costs and improving the delivery of care. At the federal level, a presidentially appointed National Health Board would interpret rules about coverage and benefits, allocate limits on premium growth among the alliances, and establish a system for monitoring how well plans, providers, and the system as a whole are performing. The states would not only establish the alliances but also retain authority to regulate insurance, certify plans, and license health professionals.

The Health Security plan would affect nearly every aspect of the health care system. Without trying to cover every feature, I want to explore the core elements in more detail in order to help explain how they fit together—and why they work.

The Logic of Comprehensive Coverage

Although hardly anyone opposes universal coverage or comprehensive benefits in principle, many have doubts whether they are workable or affordable in practice. But much as other industrialized countries provide comprehensive coverage for all their citizens, so can the United States—if we use reform to insist on mutual responsibility for payment and clear accountability for the costs.

The Health Security plan requires universal participation in the interest not only of fairness but also of lower cost to the community at large. Lack of coverage doesn't prevent money from being spent on medical care; most of the sick and injured still receive treatment, albeit less adequate care often at a later and more costly stage of illness. If insurance is voluntary, some who are healthy gamble on their good fortune and then throw themselves on the compassion of others in the hour of their need. A decent society will not leave them to suffer, but a prudent nation will have asked them beforehand to share in the cost. Most of us willingly pay for fire protection even though our house may never burn. Similarly, we must pay for health coverage to support the health care in our communities that may someday save our lives.

Universal participation makes coverage more affordable for three distinct reasons. First, it reduces the number of free riders who force others to pay more in taxes and medical bills for the uncompensated care that they (or their employees) receive. So while universal coverage provides protection to the uninsured, it also protects the rest of the community from hidden cost shifts.

Second, universal coverage reduces the problem of adverse selection that afflicts a voluntary system. If coverage is voluntary, the individuals and small groups that purchase it will include disproportionate numbers of people with high expected costs, and the resulting higher premiums will then deter many other lower-risk people who otherwise might have bought insurance.

Third, a universal system has lower administrative costs. It obviates the need of hospitals for elaborate admitting and eligibility verification procedures to protect against unpaid bills, and it cuts the administrative cost of insurance itself by eliminating functions performed in a voluntary system, such as screening out the sick.

Universal participation also makes it feasible to remove some of the most egregious limitations on coverage in the current system. Under a voluntary system, some people will wait until they get sick to buy insurance; that is one reason why insurers restrict coverage of preexisting conditions. A universal system can fairly

Covered Benefits

• Hospital services, including bed and board, routine care, therapeutics, laboratory and diagnostic and radiology services and professional services
• Emergency services
• Services of health professionals delivered in professional offices, clinics, and other sites
• Clinical preventive services
• Mental health and substance-abuse services: inpatient mental health treatment, up to thirty days per episode and sixty days per year; psychotherapy up to thirty visits per year
• Family planning services
• Pregnancy-related services
• Hospice care during the last six months of life
• Home health care, including skilled nursing care, physical, occupational, and speech therapy, prescribed social services and home-infusion therapy after an acute illness to prevent institutional care
• Extended care services, including inpatient care in a skilled nursing home or rehabilitation center following an acute illness for up to 100 days each year
• Ambulance services
• Outpatient laboratory and diagnostic services
• Outpatient prescription drugs and biologicals, including insulin
• Outpatient rehabilitation services including physical therapy and speech pathology to restore function or minimize limitations as a result of illness or injury

- Durable medical equipment, prosthetic and orthotic devices
- Routine ear and eye examinations every two years
- Eyeglasses for children under age eighteen
- Dental care for children under age eighteen

Additional Benefits in the year 2001

- Preventive dental care for adults
- Orthodontia if necessary to prevent reconstructive surgery for children
- Expanded coverage for mental health and substance abuse treatment

prohibit such limitations because no one can put off paying for insurance until the moment they need it.

Comprehensiveness of health coverage, like universality, reflects an interest in efficiency as well as equity. Benefits packages vary in their scope of coverage and extent of cost-sharing. The scope of benefits covered in the guaranteed package in the Clinton Health Security plan corresponds to the list in good corporate health plans today (see chart, above). The benefits package, however, is especially comprehensive on the "front end" (primary and preventive care) and on the "back end" (there are no lifetime or annual limits on hospital or physician coverage).

Broad benefits in these areas reflect two central objectives of reform: preventive care and security. The plan encourages a shift toward preventive care by guaranteeing coverage of a basic list of clinical preventive services of proven efficacy, such as immunizations and specific screening tests, without any copayment. And it eliminates the annual and lifetime limitations on hospital and physician coverage as well as other exclusions buried in the "fine print" of insurance contracts that expose many families to catastrophic costs and financial ruin.

Restricting both the "front" and "back" ends of health coverage often produces counterproductive results and savings that prove to be illusory. Limits on primary and preventive care lead to avoidable illness, costly delays in treatment, and greater use of emergency rooms. And when coverage runs out, many people facing catastrophic health costs end up at public hospitals or with unpaid bills, and the taxpayers or privately insured pay for their care anyway.

While its coverage is broad in scope, the Health Security plan does not eliminate all patient cost-sharing. Rather, it provides for three types of cost-sharing that correspond to the principal modes of coverage in the market today. For *fee-for-service coverage*, the cost-sharing would be in the middle range of private plans. There would be deductibles of $200 per individual and $400 per family, with 20 percent coinsurance for physician and hospital care, up to a maximum out-of-pocket cost of $1,500 per individual and $3,000 per family. Prescription drugs would carry a separate $250 deductible and 20 percent cost-sharing, up to a maximum out-of-pocket expense of $1,000.

For *HMO coverage* (the low cost-sharing option), there would be no deductibles, nor would there be any coinsurance on hospital care. The Health Security plan does, however, call for a $10 copayment per physician visit, which is higher than many HMOs charge today. The HMO copayment for drugs would be $5 per prescription.

The third type of plan, a *combined* structure, offers

the low HMO cost-sharing when patients use providers within the network but requires the higher fee-for-service cost-sharing level when patients use providers outside the network. This is the arrangement used by preferred provider networks.

The level of benefits in the Health Security plan is squarely in the mainstream; the plan does not ask Americans to accept a lower standard of coverage or offer them only minimal protection if they lose a job or get divorced.

Several other proposals for reform, however, call for only minimal coverage, restricted to catastrophic costs or a mere "barebones" package. Some conservatives believe that Americans are "overinsured" and want to use tax policy and health reform to encourage high deductibles and copayments as a method of cost containment. That approach, however, will not only fail to guarantee security; it is also unlikely to control costs effectively for the most basic of reasons: Most people won't accept it.

If national reform provides only minimal coverage, the great majority of Americans will obtain supplementary insurance. Nine out of ten Medicare beneficiaries today have supplementary coverage either through a private Medigap policy or Medicaid. These supplementary benefits typically reduce patient cost-sharing and generate higher rates of physician and hospital use *under Medicare*. Thus widespread supplementation raises costs in the basic insurance program, defeating the economic rationale of the coverage limits. A new federal program with high cost-sharing and limited benefits for the under–sixty-five population would just repeat the same mistake. Most Americans would get extra coverage from their employers, and the very poor would retain the broader coverage of Medicaid. With only

low-wage workers facing the benefit limits, there would
be little effective discipline on costs. A reformed system
is far more likely to control costs by making a single
health plan accountable for comprehensive coverage
than by dividing coverage between a minimal basic
package and widespread supplementation.

This is the broader lesson of integrated health plans.
Many coverage restrictions that developed under traditional insurance do not make sense as rules for the
emerging health care system. Since traditional insurers
have not had contracts with providers, much less control over them, they have been unable to allocate resources among different types of services or achieve
savings by managing services more efficiently. To control
costs, they have often simply excluded services—such as
primary and preventive care, outpatient drugs, and
home health services—that can reduce overall costs if
managed properly. Integrated health plans do precisely
that, substituting ambulatory for inpatient care and
managing the full range of services to provide broader
coverage more economically.

The new paradigm of integrated health care requires a
change in thinking about coverage. Under a more integrated system, arbitrary limits on coverage by type of
service or provider often get in the way of cost-effective
treatment; coverage without those restrictions yields better treatment at lower cost. Genuine savings in health
care come not from trying to shift risks to individuals,
but from placing those risks on organizations that can
manage them and be held clearly accountable for both
costs and quality.

A uniform benefits package among competing plans
facilitates that clear accountability. If each plan offers a
different package, the myriad complex variations make
it difficult for consumers to make clear-cut price com-

parisons. A uniform package enables consumers to compare apples with apples and thereby encourages plans to compete on price. Consumers will also feel more confident about choosing a lower-cost plan if they know there are no hidden exclusions.

Requiring plans to offer a uniform package does not prevent them from offering other benefits in supplementary packages (although those must be fully priced to include utilization effects on the basic plan). The required package sets a common reference point that is essential not only for price competition but also for determining rights and obligations. If a national guarantee of universal coverage is to have any meaning, there needs to be a national standard. All parties involved must know what is included in the coverage that citizens have a right to expect, plans have an obligation to provide, and government has a pledge to guarantee.

Some reform proposals accept the need for a standard benefits package but, rather than spell it out in legislation, assign the responsibility to an administrative board. The political appeal of this approach is obvious. Defining a benefits package is inevitably contentious. However, if the American people are to evaluate any proposal, they must know what the benefits are. Moreover, no one will be able to determine how much coverage will cost without knowing what coverage includes. Some critics have charged that the Clinton program vests too much power in government bureaucracies. The National Health Board set up under the Clinton plan, however, would only interpret the benefits package. Other proposals give an administrative board authority to *determine* the standard package, which would make the board far more powerful. In another area as well—the role and power of the purchasing alliances—conservative alternatives ostensibly aimed at reducing costs and bureaucracy actually increase them.

The Role of the Health Alliances

No aspect of reform is so poorly understood and so critical to its success as the broad-based purchasing alliances of the Health Security plan. Without the alliances, it will not be possible to shift the choice of health plans from employers to consumers, to restore genuine community rating, and to achieve effective reform of the insurance system.

The Clinton plan calls for two types of purchasing alliances. Regional health alliances would cover all employees of firms with fewer than 5,000 workers, public employees, part-time workers, the unemployed, and other individuals outside the labor force—in all, more than 80 percent of the population under age sixty-five. The regional alliances would thus constitute a pool covering the vast majority of Americans at community rates. Corporations with more than 5,000 employees, as well as some multiemployer plans of similar size established through collective bargaining, would be eligible to establish their own corporate health alliances. Corporate alliances would still have to provide their employees at least the guaranteed benefits package and a choice among the three types of plans, but they would not be eligible for any federal subsidies and would pay an assessment equal to 1 percent of payroll. (The assessment goes for medical education and public health and makes up for the cost advantages that companies enjoy in running a self-contained pool without the unemployed, the retired, and the poor.) Large corporations could opt into the regional alliances on an initially risk-adjusted basis, a provision designed to offset the costs of large companies with many older workers. If they came in, they would become eligible for the 7.9 percent cap on contributions on a graduated basis beginning after four years.

The regional alliances would have the responsibility of ensuring that all eligible people in an area were enrolled in a health plan (people who didn't sign up would be enrolled when they showed up for medical care). The alliances would disseminate information about plans and run the open enrollment, collect funds from employers and individuals and disburse them to plans, and make the risk adjustment in payments to plans according to procedures set down by the National Health Board.

The Clinton plan requires regional alliances to offer at least one traditional fee-for-service plan covering "any willing provider" as well as any other plan that meets the terms of participation. (However, the Health Security Act prohibits states from requiring that *all* plans pay any willing provider, which would make HMOs and provider networks impossible to organize.) The terms include the basic requirements for fair competition: open enrollment, community rating, no preexisting condition exclusions, reporting of data on the quality of care, and no discrimination against consumers on the basis of race, gender, disability, health status, or other characteristics. Alliances could exclude a health plan if it did not observe these practices, failed to provide the benefits, or flunked a state's minimum quality standards. In addition, if a plan's bid exceeded the average premium by more than 20 percent, alliances would not be required to offer it—a provision aimed at giving alliances bargaining leverage with high-cost plans.

With an average of more than 80 percent of the under–sixty-five population in a region, the alliances' inclusive membership would enable them to recreate the broad pooling of risk that has been lost in recent decades as the insurance industry has segmented the market, cherry-picked the healthy groups, and denied coverage to many small firms and individuals or charged them unaffordable rates. In addition, the alliances would open up more options to millions of consumers, including many of the insured who have never had access to any plan except the one given them by their employer. And because the alliances would represent so large a pool, few if any health plans or groups of providers would be able to bypass them or offer unfavorable rates. From the plans' standpoint, the alliances would be the point of access to the overwhelming majority of middle-class patients—not just the poor and the unemployed. This is vital to ensuring that the people participating in the alliances get the widest possible options at the best prices.

Health alliances can succeed only if the insurers must go through them to reach the market in the region. If health plans are able to sign up individuals directly, they are as certain to sign up the best risks as water is to roll downhill. And if plans can cut their costs by selectively enrolling healthy people rather than by managing services efficiently, competition will fail to generate real savings. Thus to make competition work, the alliances must conduct the annual open enrollment independent of any plan and risk-adjust payments to insurance plans so that there are no rewards for "cream skimming."

Some critics have charged that the alliances would be a new and unneeded "layer of bureaucracy." The alliances, however, would assume functions now performed by benefits managers, brokers, and other intermediaries. They *subtract* more administrative costs than they add, especially in the individual and small-group insurance markets, where, as I've indicated, administrative costs currently run as high as 40 cents on the premium dollar.

Ironically, the alternatives advocated by some conservatives—smaller, voluntary alliances with no required employer contributions—will actually raise costs, increase administrative overhead, and permit insurance companies to continue cherry-picking the healthy instead of refocusing their energies on lower cost and better quality. Voluntary alliances would have higher premiums because they would be left with relatively older and less healthy employee groups as well as the unemployed. Voluntary alliances would also cost more to administer because they would have to devote significant resources to marketing and could only spread their fixed costs over a smaller population. And without required employer contributions, premium collections would be less reliable.

Two proposals in Congress that call for voluntary purchasing cooperatives raise these problems. The conservative Democrats' bill, advanced by Representative Jim Cooper, would limit eligibility for its regional purchasing cooperatives to residents of an area otherwise without insurance and to firms with fewer than 100 employees. Another bill backed by Senate Republicans and introduced by Senator John Chafee calls for competing, voluntary purchasing cooperatives, also limited to employers with fewer than 100 workers. Neither proposal requires employers to contribute, though the Chafee plan envisions a mandate on individuals to buy a minimum level of insurance in the year 2005.

Both the Cooper and Chafee proposals threaten to raise premiums in the purchasing cooperatives above the levels for larger firms as a result of adverse selection. Because the proposals do not require participation in the cooperatives, the most likely to purchase coverage will be individuals or groups with relatively higher risks. And because the cooperatives are restricted to uninsured individuals and employees of small firms, they make up a pool whose costs are higher than the population in larger firms. The relationship between the size of firms in the cooperatives and average premiums is direct: The lower the cut-off point for firms, the higher the average premiums will be.

The likely concentration of high-cost populations in the smaller, voluntary purchasing cooperatives is not only a matter of fairness. If the premiums in the alliances cost more, businesses and unions will seek to get out and the cooperatives will unravel. Small businesses will not want to share in the costs of the unemployed and the poor. Moreover, some health plans may decide not to contract with these high-cost voluntary cooperatives, or the plans will offer only high rates to offset the risks. As a result, voluntary cooperatives may not be able to ensure that their members can obtain affordable coverage. Competition among the cooperatives would only make the problem worse: To reduce risks, cooperatives—like insurers today—would have an incentive to avoid covering high-cost groups.

Some critics suggest that purchasing alliances are unnecessary because their aims can be achieved by insurance market reforms, such as community rating. However, if employers can still self-insure, the "community" being rated will consist of people left out of larger and healthier employee groups, and rates will inevitably be higher. And without the alliances to manage the competition and run the enrollment, insurance plans will continue to compete by dodging high-cost populations. Moreover, this would be a system of employer, not consumer, choice of health plan—with all the attendant problems of employer-sponsored insurance in an age of managed care (see above, Chapter Five). And with no purchasing alliances, small employers, the self-employed, and other individuals will continue to see a staggering share of the premium dollar eaten up by insurance overhead costs.

By requiring the participation of all employers with fewer than 5,000 employees in a single pool, the Clinton plan creates a broad, stable foundation for the alliances. Rather than being stuck with high costs, Americans who receive coverage through the alliances will benefit from their great combined purchasing power and economies of scale. Small businesses and individuals will be able to obtain health coverage on terms previously available only to the biggest companies. Conservative critics have objected that the alliances will be monopolies (or, to use the exact term, monopsonies) in their regions. However, the ultimate buyers are individual consumers; the alliances organize the competition to reorient health plans from avoiding risk to providing good care at an affordable cost. A structure for the alliances that allows insurers to cherry-pick and guarantees high premiums will raise federal subsidy costs and make it difficult to achieve universal coverage, postponing the real reform we need.

Improving the Quality of Care
In the debate over health care reform, most attention has focused on controlling costs and ensuring security and access to health care. But one of the most distinctive aspects of comprehensive reform today is its potential to improve the quality of care. In the past, health insurance and the delivery of health services were institutionally separate; indeed, public and private insurance programs were often specifically barred from interfering in medical practice.

Today, the consolidation of health insurance and health services into integrated health plans has opened up new possibilities for holding plans and providers accountable for quality and access as well as cost.

There is also growing appreciation that poor quality and high cost are related. Earlier proposals for universal coverage did not build in concern for quality because they generally assumed that spending more money for more services would bring better care. By now we should have learned to stop equating "more" with "better." Much of the excess cost in the U.S. system stems from unneeded and inappropriate care; reform that reduces such excess can raise quality and cut costs simultaneously.

To many people, reducing costs through improved quality sounds like a chimera, but the new forms of quality management in American industry start from exactly that premise. Poor quality is costly; doing things right the first time is cheaper than doing them over. Traditional quality control focuses on picking out defective products and punishing poor performers. That approach not only fails to identify the systemic causes of mistakes and poor quality; it also intimidates and inhibits employees from contributing to improve quality. The new approaches in industry emphasize learning rather than punishment. Instead of relying on surveillance and inspection, they call for close attention to the demands of customers, systematic measurement of outcomes, emulation of "best practice" models, cooperative efforts at quality improvement involving employees at every level of an organization, and continuous monitoring and correcting of performance.

The same movement is stirring in health care, attempting to reform health care from within, and the aim of the Clinton Health Security plan is to create a broader institutional framework that supports those efforts. The purpose of reform is not to impose a new regime, but to help stimulate and nurture the most auspicious changes already under way. In health care, as in other fields, traditional quality assessment emphasizes case-by-case, punitive regulation. In contrast, the Health Security plan seeks to encourage more systematic measurement of the outcomes of care and an emphasis on correcting the root problems that cause poor quality.

Inadequate knowledge about what works in health care is the critical barrier to improving care. We suffer from two kinds of ignorance, for which we need two kinds of remedy. In some areas, health professionals face uncertainty because scientific knowledge is inadequate. For that problem the only known remedy is research, and the Health Security plan provides funds for that purpose, particularly research on the outcomes of care. In other areas, both providers and consumers face uncertainty because there has been no systematic effort to obtain comparative data about how well plans and providers are performing. In principle, we could know; we just haven't tried to find out. Here we need a commitment to regular monitoring of the various dimensions of performance. The Clinton plan makes that commitment an integral part of national reform.

The Health Security plan calls for attention to six aspects of performance: *access to care*, *the appropriateness of care*, *outcomes of care*, *consumer satisfaction*, *health promotion*, and *disease prevention*. To provide comparative data on these dimensions, there must be commonly agreed upon indicators and methods. The establishment of a National Quality Management Council to choose the quality indicators and methods of collection is one of the responsibilities of the National Health Board. The resulting data will have several uses. They will be combined into an annual public report about how well health plans and providers are performing on key criteria, and the reports will be made available both to consumers to assist them in their choices and to providers to help them do a better job. The data will also be used to guide research priorities and evaluate the performance and impact of the entire reform program in order to make midcourse corrections.

Comparative value information is an idea that has come to health care only recently, but it is familiar to anyone who has opened an issue of *Consumer Reports* and checked the ratings on different products and services. To be sure, most people do not read the ratings, but to generate competition on quality, not everyone has to. Even a minority of quality-sensitive buyers can affect an entire market. Besides, the news media are scarcely likely to ignore assessments of the quality of care, especially when nearly everybody in a community has access to the same list of health plans.

The Health Security plan also calls for technical assistance to plans and providers to help them learn how to correct the causes of poor quality care. The responsibility for that assistance will belong to regional professional foundations, made up of representatives of academic health centers, health plans, health alliances, and practicing physicians and other provider groups.

Several other provisions of the Clinton plan fit into the concern for improving quality and cutting costs. The application of information technology to health care holds enormous promise not just to cut the cost of administrative transactions and eliminate duplicate testing, but to reduce errors in treatment and enable professionals and patients alike to make better decisions. The greater use of electronic information systems will also help reduce the "cost of quality" by permitting less burdensome tracking of treatments and outcomes. Computerized records, however, raise concerns about confidentiality and security. So while the Clinton plan supports advances in health care information systems, it also calls for the first national standards for confidentiality of medical information and strict penalties for breaches of privacy and security.

Another major concern of the Clinton plan is support for primary and preventive care. The plan proposes a dramatic shift in the priorities of graduate medical education away from specialization toward primary care, and it provides greater support for training of advanced-practice nurses. The plan also seeks to increase rewards for primary care in Medicare's payment system. Inadequate numbers of primary care providers represent an obstacle to providing appropriate care and coordinated services—especially in communities with the greatest needs.

Protecting the Vulnerable

The approach of the Health Security plan to ensuring access for underserved and vulnerable populations is similar to its approach to improving the quality of care. The plan relies on both a general framework for achieving accountability and a series of targeted efforts aimed at overcoming barriers to good health care.

The general framework has been implicit in much of the previous discussion. Both the health alliances and health plans have responsibilities to ensure that underserved communities and vulnerable groups have access. While the alliances must ensure enrollment, the plans must ensure that members receive appropriate services. Access to care and consumer satisfaction are two of the criteria for regular evaluations of health plans, and the quality management program is specifically responsible for obtaining representative data on populations at risk of inadequate care.

This approach builds in a set of obligations missing from traditional insurance programs like Medicaid. Medicaid provides coverage for many low-income people, but until the recent development of managed care in Medicaid, the program did not vest any health care organization with responsibility for providing access to care. While beneficiaries have had a Medicaid card, many have often been unable to find a doctor because Medicaid payment levels have been so low that no physician will take them, or none is available in their area. Fee-for-service Medicaid could not hold any particular providers accountable for failing to serve the poor or the disabled. In contrast, under the alliances, health plans would be contractually obligated to provide care for all their subscribers. If vulnerable groups did not receive care, they would have not merely a general complaint but specific contractual rights.

Many advocacy groups for the poor are nonetheless skeptical about competition and private health plans. Their experience has taught them that the health care market works poorly for the underserved; this has undoubtedly been true. But in several critical respects, the Health Security plan departs sharply from the status quo. Today, health care services in low-income areas are precariously financed because so many of their patients are uninsured or reimbursed at Medicaid levels. By covering the entire population and integrating Medicaid beneficiaries into private plans, the Clinton plan puts providers in low-income areas on a more stable, secure footing.

The risk-adjustment system provides further benefit to the providers who care for low-income and vulnerable populations. Today, such providers generally receive lower payment even though they take care of people with some of the most severe problems. After reform, health plans will receive more for enrollees that generate higher costs. To be sure, the methods of risk adjustment are far from perfect. Risk adjustment, however, provides a mechanism for targeting funds where the needs are greatest. It may prove to be far more effective in channeling resources to populations in need than grant programs that depend on discretionary government funding.

Advocacy groups have also worried that under reform the community health centers, public hospitals, and other providers of care in low-income communities might be locked out of private health plans, lose their patients, and face worse financial woes than they do today. The Clinton plan addresses those concerns in several ways. First, for at least a five-year transitional period, the federal government will designate qualifying organizations providing care to vulnerable groups as essential community providers. Health plans will either have to enter into contracts with these providers or pay them on a fee-for-service basis, unless they can demonstrate they have adequate services available in the same communities.

The Health Security plan also offers funds to help community providers establish their own networks and plans as well as to support development of adequate service capacity to provide care in underserved areas. Over the period between 1995 and 2000, the Clinton plan allocates a total of $15 billion in new federal funds for public health initiatives; many of these initiatives support health care in both rural and urban underserved communities. These include grants to community and migrant health centers, support for school-based health

services, and an expansion of the National Health
Service Corps, which awards scholarship aid to medical
students in return for later service in designated shortage
areas.

In addition, the Health Security plan is the source of
an indirect windfall to state and local governments that
are now funding public clinics and hospitals. Except for
illegal immigrants, the uninsured now receiving those
services will gain private coverage. As a result, the
Health Security plan will free up approximately $65 bil-
lion in state and local health spending between 1995
and 2000. These funds could be variously used to cut
taxes, to provide supplementary services (such as trans-
portation) not covered under the guaranteed benefit
package, and to strengthen community health activities.

Keeping Coverage Affordable

Besides ensuring access for the underserved, any health
care reform plan has to ensure that health coverage is affordable to low-income Americans and to those who do
not receive a full employer contribution because they
have lost their jobs, work only part-time, or are retired
but not yet eligible for Medicare. Providing for people in
each of these situations poses an enormous challenge.

The Clinton plan provides discounts on the family
share of the premium to the poor and near-poor—
specifically, to people with incomes below 150 percent
of the poverty level. In 1993 the poverty line for a family of four was close to $15,000; thus on a sliding scale,
families would be eligible for discounts that phased out
just above $22,000 annual income. No one, poor or
otherwise, would pay more than 3.9 percent of income
for the family share of the premium.

The Health Security plan also protects the unemployed and part-time workers from unaffordable de-

mands to make up for unpaid employer contributions—that is, the share of the premium no employer ever paid because the head of a family did not work full-time for the entire year. First of all, if a couple or family had one full-time worker, no other family member would need to make up unpaid employer contributions for periods of unemployment or part-time work. One full-time worker per family (or two half-time workers) would earn a family the right to a credit from the regional alliance for a full 80 percent employer contribution toward the family premium.

Second, people who were unemployed or working part-time would be liable for the unpaid employer share only if they had income from interest, dividends, rent, capital gains, and other nonwage sources or made a lot of money when they did work (more than $5,000 a month). For example, suppose you were single and worked half-time. Under the Clinton plan, employers would pay a pro-rated amount for part-time workers to the regional alliance. As a half-time employee, your firm would pay half the employer contribution for a single worker (an average of $773 a year or $64 a month). You would owe the remaining half of the employer share on the basis of a sliding scale to the extent you had unearned income or your wages as a part-time worker exceeded $5,000 a month. If you were unemployed part of the year, unemployment compensation would not be counted toward this total. Discounts for the 80-percent employer share would phase out at 250 percent of poverty. Responsibility for administering these discounts would belong to the alliances.

Early retirees would derive particular benefit from the Clinton plan. Like everyone else, early retirees between the ages of fifty-five and sixty-five would be eligible to purchase a community-rated premium through the alliances; community rating is especially valuable to early retirees because of their age and frequency of chronic medical problems. If they met the requirements for Social Security by working ten years before retiring, the federal subsidy pool would also pick up the 80 percent employer share for retirees until they became eligible for Medicare at age sixty-five. These provisions affecting millions of Americans in the hiatus before Medicare eligibility are especially important today because rising costs and new accounting rules have led many companies to eliminate long-established health benefits for early retirees.

Ultimately, for all Americans, the affordability of coverage will depend not so much on any of these provisions as on our success in controlling the overall cost of health care. For we won't be able to afford helping those least able to pay themselves unless we put the health system on an economically sustainable and fiscally sound basis.

CHAPTER 7

FINANCING
THE PLAN

The ultimate tests of health care reform will be the quality of health care and the health of the American people. However, the first hurdle any plan must cross is financial: Can it control costs? Does it provide adequate financing for coverage? Does it protect the fiscal integrity of government and economic needs of businesses and families?

The Clinton plan has been developed in extraordinary detail to address many of the specific questions affecting families and businesses in different situations, the array of current government programs, and the transition to new financing arrangements. Behind the multitude of details, however, stand a few central ideas that represent the plan's basic strategy for containing costs and financing coverage. Understanding that strategy is vital to grasping the overall logic of reform.

Cap Globally, Act Locally

The dual reliance on competition and premium caps is the defining feature of the Health Security plan's strategy of cost containment. The strategy's first defense against rising costs is the system of purchasing alliances, incentives for cost-conscious consumer choice, and competing plans paid per capita for their enrollment. The strategy's second line of defense is a cap on the growth of average premiums in the health alliances. Some may ask, "If competition works, why bother with caps?" For the same reason that an engineer designs a plane with a backup engine or a car with an emergency brake: Designing in redundancy helps avoid failure.

Redundancy makes particular sense when there are limits to the principal mechanism of cost containment. Not every region will have vigorously competing plans, and even in areas with the potential for competition, health care providers may successfully thwart it, as they have through much of this century. The purchasing alliances and relevant government agencies might also fall under the control of provider interests; again, a long history suggests "provider capture" is a serious risk. Federally legislated caps on average alliance premiums thus represent a kind of political insurance policy. And in an industry long accustomed to rapidly rising costs, expectations are a force in their own right. The caps announce a new era.

The competitive system and the premium caps also serve another less obvious function: the decentralization of risk. Through the Medicare program, the federal government has effectively assumed the risk for health costs of the elderly. And because it has assumed the risk, it has developed increasingly intrusive microregulations aimed at controlling it. The advent of prospective hospital payment under Medicare in the 1980s was a step toward decentralization because it put hospitals at risk for costs per admission. As providers share more risk, there is less need to regulate them to control costs. The Clinton plan takes the decentralization of risk and decision making much farther. The system of payment places the risk for comprehensive coverage on private health plans, giving the plans full latitude to allocate and manage resources and negotiate prices with providers. If premiums in a region go up faster than an allowed amount, the Health Security plan focuses risk on the plans and the providers that have raised rates the most.

Under the Clinton plan, the caps apply not to the premiums of individual health plans but to an alliance's weighted-average premium (the average of all premiums weighted according to the share of enrollment in the various plans). Federal legislation would set a growth rate for premiums for covered benefits for the country as a whole, and the National Health Board would adjust that rate for specific alliances depending on demographic changes and other factors. Alliances could meet their targets without any enforcement of caps as competition held down premium increases of individual plans or as consumers switched out of high-cost plans, thereby dragging down the average. If, however, health plans' bids threatened to push an alliance's average over the allowable growth, the federal government would deny full rate increases to the plans seeking the biggest jumps and require the plans to pass on those rate reductions to their providers. Thus the premium caps achieve much the same effect as the global budgets for physician spending in the German health care system, except on a more comprehensive level.

The costs of health care vary considerably from one state to another. Some of this variation is due to differences in wage levels and other economic conditions, some to the level of insurance coverage. Much of it, however, reflects different patterns of health care, such as variations in hospital use that appear to be related to the ratio of hospital beds to people in a region. Under the Health Security plan, the premium caps set at the outset of reform would reflect historic costs in an area. However, the plan calls for a commission to report back to Congress with recommendations for a method for gradually reducing differences in premiums that are due to variations in patterns of practice. Over time, the pressure to control costs should be greatest in areas with the most costly practice patterns.

One little understood function of the caps is to reduce windfall profits to the health care industry from universal coverage. Today, provider rates and insurance premiums reflect the cost of unpaid bills left by the uninsured. After universal coverage, unless rates come down, providers would receive a windfall. In theory, competition should force providers to give up that bonanza, but to count on perfectly efficient markets would be foolhardy. In other countries, the advent of universal insurance has been accompanied by a reduction in payment rates to providers since they no longer bear the costs of charity care. The Health Security plan, however, does not include any general provider price regulation and consequently cannot use that approach. A special tax might recapture windfalls, but many groups are suspicious of the possible long-term use of such a tax. So to avoid windfalls, the method for calculating initial premium caps for the alliances pulls out the current cost of uncompensated care and sets a cap for the first year on the assumption that services for the previously uninsured are paid at average costs. With no premium caps, it is likely that health care reform would begin with a costly expansionary spurt.

Much of the controversy over the caps concerns the desirability of any spending limitation. As one might suppose, providers and insurers alike are strongly opposed to budget limits and have raised public anxieties about the prospect that health plans would run out of money during the year and be unable to provide care—as if plans do not already have to budget their expenditures based on income they receive from premiums set in advance of a year.

A second set of objections has less to do with the caps themselves than with the level of growth projected under the Clinton plan. Some critics have challenged the plan's realism, saying it assumes unrealistic savings. But the plan still assumes significant growth in health expenditures and the targets it sets are, by international standards, scarcely severe.

Until 1996, the Clinton plan assumes that expenditures will rise at currently projected rates. Then, as states carry out reform beginning in 1996, the Clinton plan would have two effects on expenditures working in opposite directions. Expanded coverage would raise spending by about 8 percent, while the purchasing alliances and competition, backed up by regional premiums caps, would cut the rate of increase in per capita costs. Initially, the effect of expanded coverage would predominate; by the year 2000, however, national health expenditures would be about one half of 1 percent of GDP less than under current policies. Thus the plan does not project any reduction in spending from current levels. National health expenditures would rise from 14.3 percent in 1993 to 16.9 percent by the year 2000. Considering that the average in industrialized countries is 7.9 percent and growing much more slowly than in the U.S., 16.9 percent is hardly austere. This is not a rationing plan. We would have "savings" only be-

cause current policies would lead U.S. health spending
to rise to 17.5 percent of GDP or more by the year 2000
if we did nothing.

The plan does call for cutting the growth rate in
spending for covered benefits from around 9 percent annually at the beginning of the 1990s to about half that
level between 1996 and 2000.[1] Under the alliances, two
distinct kinds of changes will be at work to achieve that
reduction. Besides moderating the underlying growth
rate, reform also generates one-time savings from consolidation of the small-group insurance market, consumer switching out of high-cost plans, a uniform
claims form, and other changes. It is the combination of
ongoing and one-time savings that will permit reducing
the growth rate in per capita costs to levels approaching
general inflation by late in the 1990s. The Clinton plan
also achieves a corresponding slowdown in the growth
of Medicare costs through specific reductions in future
payment increases.

Some observers have been skeptical that the U.S.
could ever undertake any general limitation on health
spending because it is such a fundamental departure

---

1. As of late 1993, the rise of health care *prices* and insurance *premiums* seems to have subsided to between 5 and 6 percent, approaching the administration's target for 1996. Thus some say the
caps are unnecessary because the "fever" of health care inflation has
already broken. However, while price and premium increases have
slowed down, overall health care expenditures rose 10.2 percent in
1993 and are projected to grow at double-digit rates in 1994. Previous history suggests the slowdown in prices and premiums is tempo-
rary and misleading. The same argument that costs were already
slowing—even the same metaphor of a "fever" breaking—was used
in the late 1970s, when the industry was haunted by the specter of
federal hospital cost containment, and again in the early 1980s, when
Margaret Heckler, then Secretary of Health and Human Services,
prematurely declared victory over health care inflation. Without a
cure for the systemic "infection," the fever will not go away.

from practices in our economy. But government already accounts for four of every ten dollars spent on health care; the lesson of recent history is that the government cannot really control the costs of the care it sponsors without more comprehensive cost containment. Out of concern about the federal deficit, support has grown in Congress for an "entitlement cap" that would limit Medicare spending, and a cap might well pass even in the absence of health care reform. But if there are no corresponding caps on private health spending, the limits on Medicare will likely result in a shift of costs to the same private sector that advocates of entitlement caps are presumably trying to protect from higher taxes. Conservatives who are serious about capping federal health costs cannot escape the logic of comprehensive spending restraint.

Expenditure limits force us to confront how much we spend for health care; that in itself will be a crucial step. A key source of high costs in the United States is their fragmentation and obscurity. Other industrial countries with national health insurance have lower health costs partly because of the higher visibility of their expenditures. To be sure, consolidated financing and global budgets provide the leverage for cost control. But fiscal arrangements not only control money; they also help clarify choices and focus opposition. In the United States, health care reform not only requires a change in incentives and organization; it requires *fiscal clarification* as well.

Reform helps to achieve that clarity in several different ways. At the national level, the federal government would set an overall growth rate for spending on benefits covered in the guaranteed package. (The cap does not, however, affect employer-paid benefits or other private coverage beyond the guaranteed package or other private spending for health care.) At the individual level, when choosing a plan, consumers would have to decide how much to spend on premiums beyond their employer or government contribution. And in between, at the regional level, the alliances would clarify how much health coverage cost in one area compared to others. The linkage of employer contributions to average alliance premiums creates a direct employer stake in regional costs.

This regional stake in costs is another distinctive feature of the Health Security plan. There is no such regional interest in the costs of the Medicare program. For example, employers and employees in Rochester, New York, do not pay lower Medicare taxes, nor do the elderly in Rochester pay lower Medicare premiums, even though Rochester's health care purchasers and planners have held down medical costs for all residents, including the elderly, far below the national average. Under the Health Security plan, in contrast, average premiums in the Rochester area alliance would be lower, and both families and employers would benefit accordingly. Except for low-income families and employers that hit the cap on their contributions, people and firms in regions with higher premiums would pay more; the alliance approach would literally bring home the cost to the community of excess expansion of hospitals and other health care facilities. If, on the other hand, reform were to nationalize health costs as Medicare does, this regional accountability would be lost, and the federal government would be engaged in a tug of war with local interests, which would continue to have an incentive to overbuild facilities and pass on the costs to the rest of the country.

As the Health Security plan gives states and regions a stake in controlling costs, so it gives them the flexibility to address the problem according to local preferences and decisions. The plan gives the states the power to determine governance of the alliances, though it requires that the alliance boards represent the purchasers—employers and consumers—rather than providers or insurers. The alliances would have authority to negotiate rate schedules for fee-for-service care with provider representatives, to use financial incentives to encourage plans in underserved areas, and to negotiate with health plans over the quality of service they provide. States would have the option of collapsing fee-for-service coverage in the alliances into a single prospectively budgeted plan. They would also have the latitude to use all-payer rate setting and health planning or to rely on more strictly market-based incentives. And if a state preferred a single-payer system, it could adopt one, as long as it provided universal coverage with the same benefits and kept spending within the budget caps.

Today, the organization of medical practice, hospitals, and other aspects of the health care system is substantially different across the country; the Clinton plan does not require either states or private-sector providers to follow a single model. Indeed, the program gives the states more flexibility than they have now. Many states have been experimenting with policies to control costs and expand access, and all are struggling with out-of-control Medicaid budgets. But federal law has severely restricted the states' ability to make health policy. For important Medicaid innovations, the states generally need a federal waiver; Medicare is virtually off-limits. The Employee Retirement and Income Security Act (ERISA) bars the states from regulating employee health benefit plans, even though the states have authority to regulate health insurance. The courts have interpreted ERISA to mean that state insurance laws apply only when employers buy coverage from insurance companies, not when they self-fund their benefits. As a result, more employers have self-insured, and the states have lost the capacity to reform health care finance. Curiously enough, therefore, national reform requires, in some respects, that the federal government deregulate the states.

Under the Health Security plan, all but the very largest private employee groups would receive coverage through a state's alliances; so too would current Medicaid recipients. The states would even have the option to integrate Medicare into the alliances as long as they provided beneficiaries with full guarantees of equal or better coverage. So while the Clinton plan creates a national framework for financing and benefits, it devolves more authority downward to states and regions in addition to decentralizing risk to private plans and providers. By decentralizing authority, the Health Security plan builds in protections for geographic diversity; by decentralizing risk, it builds in fiscal protections that none of the traditional entitlement programs have had.

Financing the Public Share

Before the public release of the Clinton plan, most Americans expected it would call for a general tax increase. The plan would certainly be far easier to understand if it simply raised taxes to pay for all new expenditures. However, it would also be hard to justify or pass such a program. Instead, the plan finances new federal costs primarily by redirecting funds from growth that would otherwise take place in existing health programs.

The key to the financing of the Clinton plan is a concept familiar mainly to fiscal experts: the baseline. The baseline is the projection of costs under current law and current trends. For Medicare, Medicaid, and other federal health programs, the baseline is increasing at about three times the rate of inflation. Thus federal spending forecasts already assume sharply higher costs for current programs. Instead of simply accepting these projected increases and then raising more money on top of them, the Clinton plan makes specific changes in federal health programs to reduce their rate of growth. It then uses the money saved to help pay for new initiatives as they are phased in. Overall, reductions in future outlays for current programs account for 57 percent of the sources of funds for new initiatives.

The reductions take several different forms. To bring Medicare's growth in costs down from three times inflation to twice inflation, the plan cuts future payment increases for providers. It also requires that the most affluent elderly—those with incomes over $100,000—pay a larger share of their premiums for Medicare Part B (primarily coverage of physician services). Both Medicare and Medicaid include "disproportionate share payments" to providers, which were originally supposed to help institutions that bear heavy costs for treating the uninsured. As universal coverage is phased in, the justification for these payments will diminish and, consequently, they can be phased down. And because Medicaid beneficiaries will receive coverage through plans in the alliances (where growth in premiums is capped), Medicaid costs will grow less rapidly after reform than under current projections. Slower growth of premiums will also yield savings in federal employee health benefits.

New revenues supply the remaining federal funds. The plan includes an increase in tobacco taxes (75 cents a pack on cigarettes and an equivalent amount on other forms of tobacco); the 1 percent of payroll assessment on large corporations that run their own health alliances; and a partial recapture of savings to companies benefiting from lower health insurance costs for early retirees. Each of these levies has a justification in its own right. Higher tobacco taxes discourage smoking, especially among the young, and help pay for the health costs of the cancer, heart disease, and other ill effects generated by smoking. The payroll assessment on corporate alliances falls on companies that will be relieved of the current cost shift from the uninsured as well as the future costs of the unemployed and the poor in the regional health alliances. The recapture tax for early retiree health costs will affect companies receiving substantial, long-term relief from the Clinton plan's retiree coverage. For the first three years after introduction of the early retiree benefit, the plan requires such companies to give back half of their savings to the federal government.

The Clinton plan does not cut back the tax advantages of employer-paid health insurance, as other plans in Congress do. There is no limit on the tax deductibility or exclusion from an employee's taxable income of employer contributions for the guaranteed benefit package. Employer contributions for additional benefits will remain tax-preferred until 2004; by then the guaranteed package will have been expanded, and the impact of the change will be small. Under the Clinton plan, employees would no longer be able to pay medical expenses with before-tax dollars in so-called "cafeteria" plans. On the other hand, the Clinton plan extends new tax benefits to private long-term care insurance.

The new expenditures under the Clinton plan fall into two groups. One set consists of benefits to the elderly and disabled; these consist primarily of the expansion of Medicare to include prescription drug coverage and the new program to support long-term care in the home. These initiatives are projected to cost $123 billion over the period between 1996 and the year 2000. Through the year 2000, other provisions of the plan will almost exactly offset those costs by reducing outlays for existing Medicare coverage by $124 billion.

The second set of initiatives ensures universal coverage and strengthens complementary public health programs. The primary governmental cost for universal coverage consists of the funds for alliances to provide premium discounts to employers, low-income families, and the unemployed. The cost of these discounts will be shared between the federal government and the states. Each state's share will depend on its current cost for the Medicaid program; under the Clinton plan, states would be required to maintain the level of that support, adjusted for the future growth of health costs. Like the federal government, however, the states would see lower obligations because the capped increases in the alliances will be less than under the current Medicaid system. New federal costs will also be offset by reductions in Medicaid costs ($89 billion)—because the alliances will cover many of Medicaid's current beneficiaries—and by reductions in Medicare costs ($22 billion)—because alliance plans will become the "primary" payers for Medicare beneficiaries who work full-time.

Over the five years from 1996 to 2000, the net new federal cost for subsidies will be $151 billion (which includes a cushion of 15 percent of the gross subsidies as a precaution against changes in behavior that are hard to estimate). This is further offset by $65 billion of Medicaid savings due to reduced disproportionate share payments and slower growth of premiums in the alliances for Medicaid's residual beneficiaries, leaving a net cost of $86 billion. In addition to the premium subsidies, there are also new federal costs for tax benefits for the self-employed ($10 billion) and the public health initiatives, administrative costs, and other measures ($53 billion). Savings in other federal health programs ($40 billion) and the new tobacco and other revenues ($175 billion) more than cover these demands. Through the year 2000, according to administration estimates, the net impact on the Treasury will be to cut the deficit by $58 billion.

Some critics suggest that before enacting universal coverage, we should wait to see lower costs in existing programs. However, it will be difficult to achieve a slow-down in the costs of those programs without universal coverage. Universal coverage is the justification for eliminating disproportionate share payments. Other savings stem from the enforceable caps backing up the competitive system in the alliances; the caps, as I've indicated, pull out the cost of uncompensated care. That cannot be justified without universal coverage. If millions are still uninsured, intensified competition will lead hospitals and other providers to abandon them because the providers will no longer be able to shift costs as easily to the insured. The political consequence of failing to achieve universal coverage will, therefore, be to inhibit competition. Some of the same critics who are skeptical of the savings also object to the caps and the alliances. They would "wait and see" not just on universal coverage but on cost containment—and then use the failure to contain costs as a reason for further delaying universal coverage. This is what we have been doing for years. It is a recipe for a continuing cycle of failure, which has very large costs of its own.

Financing the Private Share
The conventional view of reform is that it comes at the expense of the private sector because of the mandate on

employers to pay a share of premiums. The Health Security plan, however, has much less of an aggregate impact on employers than is generally supposed. While the plan requires some employers to pay for health benefits for the first time, it enables a lot of firms to pay less than they now do. Today, many employers pay more than 7.9 percent of payroll for more limited coverage; few small firms can obtain good health insurance at anything like the cost under the Health Security plan. Some employers will see an immediate reduction in their benefit costs; others will see lower increases than they would without reform. In no year will the employer sector as a whole pay more than 4 percent more than it otherwise would have paid; by the end of the decade, employers collectively will pay $27 billion less than they would under current trends.

However, some firms stand to gain and others to lose because the new system will tend to spread costs more evenly among employers. Currently insuring firms—particularly those that cover whole families and have older workers and many retirees—will tend to see lower costs, while those that have provided little or no coverage will, of course, experience increases. For example, manufacturing companies, state governments, and small businesses that now provide good health benefits will generally see reduced costs for their employees. But retail firms and other low-wage service businesses, especially those that rely heavily on part-time workers, will see higher costs. The firms facing the largest increases relative to current labor costs are employers with more than 5,000 workers, such as national retailers, that now offer no insurance and low average wages.

The Clinton plan reduces costs for currently insuring employers not only by capping contributions but also by spreading the cost of families and eliminating the costs of uncompensated care. Today, firms that pay for health insurance are indirectly covering the health costs of workers at other firms that do not provide insurance. These uninsured workers leave unpaid medical bills, and hospitals and other providers shift the costs to the insured. In addition, firms that cover dependents often pay for spouses employed at other companies. Under reform, an individual employer's contribution for an employee with a family will be reduced by about one fourth because of the contributions of other employers with family workers, and the elimination of uncompensated care will cut on average about 10 percent from current premium levels. These two sources of savings will offset additional costs, such as those for part-time workers not covered by most employers today.

The net impact of these changes on firms that now insure is striking. Without reform, average annual employer premium payments per worker are projected to rise from $1,923 in 1994 to $3,086 in the year 2000; with reform, they will increase only to $2,481—a total saving of $59 billion to currently insuring employers. As a percentage of payroll, premium payments would grow from 6.8 percent to 8.2 percent without reform by the end of the decade; under reform, they will fall slightly, to 6.6 percent.

The most strenuous opposition to required employer contributions comes from small businesses that do not currently pay anything for health benefits. However, small business owners and their employees are scarcely immune from illness. Under the current insurance system, they typically pay the most for the least adequate insurance coverage because of experience rating and insurers' high administrative costs in the small-group market. The Clinton plan's health alliances give them access to a broad pool, enabling them to purchase coverage at more favorable rates. Even at full cost, the alliances help them pay less; with the discounts, they come out far ahead compared to either the insurance rates or financial risks that they and their employees now face.

Some small business owners imagine dire consequences because they think not of the comprehensive effects on labor markets and their competitors, nor of the long-run effect on the health system, but of the short-run impact as if their business alone were being asked to pay. Yet small employers survived handily in Hawaii after health benefits were required by the state, and recent studies of federal increases in the minimum wage show little adverse effect.

Moreover, economists generally agree that the costs of health insurance are ultimately borne not by firms but by workers, except for those at the minimum wage. In recent decades, the growing cost of employer-paid health insurance has not pushed up labor's share of national income; the effect, as I noted earlier, has been to depress growth in wages. Sooner or later, workers pay for health insurance even if the employer writes the check.

The ability of employers to shift costs to their workers may explain why business has historically been so ineffective at containing costs. Internationally, there is a direct relationship between the private sector's share of health spending and the level of spending. The relationship is the reverse from what employers may believe: the greater the private share the higher the costs of health care. Most employers in the U.S. have been unable to control health costs over the long term; even today, the majority are paying list price. Our system has been sustained by the illusion on the part of employees that the insurer paid the medical bill while the employer paid the insurance bill; in fact, the workers themselves have been paying all along. Although the Health Security plan maintains employer contributions, it creates much clearer incentives for cost-conscious decisions by consumers and a framework for holding providers accountable for their full performance—cost, quality, and access. This is reform in the pursuit of responsibility as well as security.

CHAPTER 8

FROM HERE TO
REFORM—AND AFTER

Reformers have been waiting for the Big Bang in health insurance for more than seventy-five years. Several times universal health coverage has seemed almost within reach, only to recede as opposing interests mobilized and windows of political opportunity closed amid wars and recessions. Perhaps a similar scenario will unfold in the 1990s. The trend of the past decade has been for Americans to lose health coverage, not to gain it. As costs rise, more employers may drop benefits, new businesses may start without any, and public programs may be cut. Greater misery is always a possibility. The negative consensus on health care could simply grow more negative without any strong and comprehensive legislation being adopted.

Yet, with perhaps typically American optimism, I don't believe that will happen. To be sure, many people

prefer the status quo to change. But the status quo is itself changing, as rising costs threaten interests great and
small. Inertia is expensive; the present is precarious.
Many people see their options shrinking. As health insurance in the current market becomes more restrictive—excluding some Americans entirely from coverage
and limiting others' choice of providers—the system itself makes new converts to the cause of reform. The result may only be political stalemate. Or, with creative
leadership, it can be a new synthesis.

The Strengths of Synthesis

A plan for universal health insurance that calls for consumer choice, competition, and regional caps on premium growth is an ideological hybrid. Like single-payer
proposals, the Clinton plan guarantees coverage to all
Americans as a right of citizenship, provides comprehensive health benefits, limits burdens according to ability to pay, and caps growth in expenditures for covered
benefits. Like more conservative proposals that emphasize competition, this approach enables Americans to receive coverage through a health plan of their own
choosing, obliges plans to compete on price and quality
for enrollment, and asks consumers to bear the marginal
cost of health plans that produce the guaranteed benefits
package at a higher premium.

On each side of the spectrum, some consider elements
of this framework to be heresy, and others simply find it
puzzling. Nonetheless, it has a coherent logic. It builds
on the experience of successful health care organizations
in the United States. It builds in flexibility for states. It
incorporates a backup system for cost containment in
case competition fails or simply isn't practical in a region.

This approach does not penalize Americans who now

have good coverage or who may want to buy extra coverage. If their employer now covers a broader set of benefits, they can continue to receive those additional benefits (with full tax advantages until 2004); supplementary packages will also be available to individuals to buy on their own. Alliances are required to offer a fee-for-service option. The Health Security plan seeks to reduce inequalities in health care, not by restricting the affluent but by giving greater security and broader choice to everyone else.

This is *inclusive* reform. It brings the uninsured, the unemployed, and the poor into a mainstream standard of coverage instead of segregating them in a separate program. Low-income families will receive discounts, based on the average premium in a region, to enable them to afford coverage through some of the same private health plans available to the middle class. The uniform guaranteed benefits package will not only reduce disparities in coverage; it will also reduce premium differences among the plans. Medicaid will cease to exist as a separate program with a lower rate of payment to doctors.

To the public at large, reform offers vital protections. It will close gaps in coverage for millions of people by eliminating annual and lifetime limitations and covering preexisting conditions, preventive services, and prescription drugs. The guarantee that coverage can never be taken away is a benefit even for those who now have good coverage but worry about its dependability. Under reform, no American need fear that losing or changing jobs might cost their family access to health care; none need fear the financial devastation suffered by many today whose coverage runs out or disappears when an insurer refuses to renew a policy. All Americans would receive comprehensive benefits, with the right to choose among different health plans competing for their favor in a framework with strong consumer protections.

Today, many employees and their families are losing options they used to have as companies substitute a single managed care plan for traditional health insurance. Under the Clinton plan, the alliances will provide the full menu of health plans available in a community. Consumers could continue to see the same doctors and other providers by enrolling in a traditional fee-for-service plan, or they could sign up for a network or HMO in which their doctor participates. The alliances shift the power of choice from employers to individual consumers. Today, the option of conventional fee-for-service insurance covering any willing provider is disappearing; the costs are becoming prohibitive in part because fee-for-service attracts older and sicker enrollees. The alliances will adjust payments to plans for differences in enrollment patterns, and they will also be able to keep down the cost of fee-for-service insurance by negotiating fee-for-service rates with providers. Thus the alliances may well preserve fee-for-service from extinction. In addition, under the Clinton plan, even HMOs will be required to offer a point-of-service plan, enabling consumers to go to a provider outside the plan, albeit at a higher copayment.

Furthermore, the Clinton plan seeks to empower consumers by giving them good information about their alternatives and enabling them to take their dollars to the plans and providers that serve them best. The point of giving choice to consumers is not just controlling costs but compelling plans and providers to be responsive to the concerns of their patients. Informed choice can thereby improve the real value Americans get from their health care.

Reform offers the promise not only of more security

but also of greater liberty. Today's health insurance system limits basic economic freedoms, preventing millions of Americans from becoming fully productive citizens. The system blocks many Americans from taking new jobs because someone in their family would lose coverage of a preexisting condition. Some employees are reluctant to start a small business of their own because they cannot obtain health insurance for their family at an affordable rate. Many recipients of public assistance stay on welfare primarily to qualify for Medicaid because the jobs available to them don't carry health benefits, and the same is true for many people with disabilities. If they wish to qualify for government health benefits, they often cannot work. But if they want to work, they often cannot find a job that provides health coverage. Firms are also less likely today to employ people with high health costs because each firm's costs depend on the health of its own employees.

By prohibiting exclusions of preexisting conditions and requiring all employers to provide health coverage, the Health Security plan eliminates both job lock and welfare lock. Community rating and discounts to small business will facilitate the formation of small businesses by people now locked into corporate jobs because of family health problems. And because the plan links employer contributions to average premiums in health alliances, it enables individual employers to hire workers with disabilities without seeing their insurance rates go up. That will reduce barriers to employment. One provision of the Clinton plan goes even further. People with disabilities will receive a tax credit for personal assistance services worth 50 percent of earnings—a major incentive to take a job. In addition, the expansion of home- and community-based long-term care will open up opportunities to go to work for many people—primarily women—who are now at home caring for an elderly parent or disabled member of their family.

All these positive effects on work, employment, and economic freedom need to be remembered amid the noisy claims of opponents that the President's plan will hurt small business and jobs. A fair assessment will show that the benefits for business and the economy outweigh the disadvantages.

Reform and the Emerging Health Care System

Twenty years ago, health insurance programs were conceivable with no controls on medical services. Such was the original framework of Medicare. But that approach is no longer plausible, as the subsequent history and growing financial burden of Medicare itself indicate. To ensure economic security to individuals, national health reform must include universal coverage. To provide economic security to the country, it must now simultaneously be a program for cost containment.

Change is already under way in health care. Health plans with their own networks of providers are gaining in enrollment, while traditional fee-for-service insurance is shrinking. In some respects, the Clinton plan builds on changes in progress; in other respects, it attempts to redirect that evolution. The distinction is crucial: It builds on the new plans and networks, but it changes the basic rules of the market and the framework of choice.

Reform will unquestionably mean major changes for the insurance industry. Under the Clinton plan, alliances will absorb functions now performed by insurance brokers, consultants, and employee benefits managers. Open enrollment, community rating, and competition on a standard benefits package will force insurance companies that have profited by cherry-picking the healthy, rather than controlling medical costs, either to adapt or to leave the field. Many observers assume that larger insurance companies will benefit. Some companies that have invested in managed care are well positioned to grow, but it is not clear that plans run by big insurance companies will become dominant.

Under the alliances, groups of providers can accept payment directly without the mediation of insurance companies. If community hospitals, groups of physicians, and other providers can create community-based health plans that effectively manage capacity, they should enjoy major competitive advantages. As well-established providers of care, they are already known and trusted in their communities and do not need to build or buy up facilities to provide service. The alliances, moreover, are the key that unlocks the market for them. Today, community-based plans are difficult to start because they need to be marketed to thousands of employers. Under reform, the regional health alliance will provide them access to virtually the entire market in their region.

Thus the alliances have major advantages for community hospitals and local physicians. Today, patients' options depend on their employers. Doctors often lose satisfied patients because of employers' decisions to change health plans. To protect their access to patients, some physicians now feel obliged to accept virtually whatever terms insurer-run networks offer them. Under reform, patients will be able to follow their doctors to the health plans in which the doctors participate. In general, patients have far more trust in their physicians than they have in insurance companies. If the doctors urge patients to choose community-based plans, those plans may well prevail.

Some insurers have said they are all in favor of insurance market reforms but oppose the alliances as an unneeded government bureaucracy. The reasons for their opposition are transparent. The alliances will confront the insurers with much stronger buyers. Moreover, many insurers are plainly threatened by the growth of integrated health plans, including the community-based networks. It is no surprise, therefore, that the Health Insurance Association of America wants the alliances to be merely voluntary for employers. That way insurers would continue to be able to cherry-pick the best risks, leaving the highest-cost groups to the alliances.

Much depends on the exact form that final federal legislation takes. If health plans are required to serve an entire region or to maintain large capital reserves, or if the criteria for certifying plans impose excessive demands upon them, community-based plans will find it hard to compete and may be forced to serve as networks within insurer-run systems. And if alliances are small and voluntary, they will become high-risk pools and be incapable of giving consumers the power of choice and good value for their money. Employer-based managed care, with all its disadvantages, will predominate.

Thus the Clinton plan has some clear-cut advantages for doctors and other providers over other proposals for reform. This approach leaves physicians with a variety of different practice options, from fee-for-service to staff-model HMOs. Although the alliances would negotiate fee-for-service rates with provider representatives, there is no all-payer fee regulation. Plans would negotiate their own payment rates with the physicians and other providers with whom they have contracts. And community-based plans could preserve the independence of local hospitals and doctors.

I do not want to suggest, however, that the medical profession will benefit economically compared to the

status quo. According to a study by two health economists, Gregory Pope and John Schneider, national
spending on physicians' services doubled in real terms
between 1980 and 1989, up from $63.1 billion to
$117.6 billion in constant 1989 dollars. Over the decade
from 1978 to 1988, they estimate that real net income—
that is, after expenses and after inflation—rose 46 percent for surgeons, 24 percent for medical specialists, and
9 percent for general and family practitioners. It seems
highly unlikely that if the U.S. had earlier adopted competition under a cap, total spending on physicians' services would have grown as fast or that surgeons would
have benefited as much. Global caps would have re-
strained the growth of physician income, and competitive health plans would probably have concentrated a
larger share of surgical procedures in fewer hands, in-
tensifying pressures on surgeons to cut fees.

Yet it is also unlikely that reform would have entirely
blocked growth in spending or spread income gains
equally among physician specialties. The surgeons' rising incomes reflect both higher profit margins (which
are vulnerable to competitive forces) and an increasing
volume of complex procedures. Surgeons are benefiting
from a technological explosion that is unlikely to quiet
down any time soon. HMO and other health plans,
moreover, will not be in a position, even under reform,
to dictate terms to doctors because they will need the
physicians' cooperation to control overall health costs.
Or, to put it another way, doctors can save money for
health plans, not just by keeping down increases in their
own fees but by conserving health care resources. And
from the health plans' standpoint, the latter may be far
more important.

A competitive system is also unlikely to threaten the
extinction of private medical practice. As they do today,

health plans will generally find it in their interest to contract with independent physicians and physician groups. Even among prepaid group practices, the group-model plans (where physician partnerships are independent of the plans) seem to have better growth prospects than do staff-model plans. As Alan Hillman and his colleagues at the University of Pennsylvania have pointed out, many HMOs now deal with an intermediate physician organization that exercises the real control over the rules and compensation packages for individual doctors. The development of a competitive system may push doctors to organize themselves into more multispecialty group practices, but the plans are unlikely to make most doctors their employees.

In areas such as California or Minnesota where there is already intense health plan competition, health care reform will not dramatically alter the conditions of medical practice. Many practitioners will find their professional work little changed from what it is today—except that all their patients will have health coverage under one plan or another. In other areas of the country like Texas, where traditional fee-for-service still reigns, the changes could be considerable (as they would be under other proposals favoring managed care). The varying response of physicians from California and Texas to the Clinton plan has reflected these differences.

As the health care system changes, so it is reshaping the political outlook of the medical profession. The development of managed care plans tends to diminish the opposition of physicians to public programs for the uninsured and to raise their anxieties about domination by business. In the nineteenth century, when they sought licensing protection from the state, doctors tended to support a stronger role for government. They became devoted to laissez faire only after their incomes rose and they began to worry that a public insurance system would deprive them of their autonomy. As the twentieth century ends, the profession appears to be reverting toward a more positive view of the state. The profession's current divisions and ambivalence may reflect the uneven extent of the current transformation of medical care.

A narrow, last-ditch defense of traditional prerogatives and the economic interests of private practice will be self-defeating. The era of limits has been long in coming; its arrival has been delayed but it is certain. Rather than struggling to maintain the status quo, physicians and other providers would be much better served by taking a positive role in bringing about change—indeed, leading it—as many have done in recent years.

It will not be easy for the physicians—or for other groups. The prospect of change raises anxieties, and the nearer change approaches, the more fearful many people become. Some of the anxiety is natural. Some of it is being stirred up by the insurance industry, insurance brokers, and other interests that stand to lose economically and have become the purveyors of panic in the crowded theater of reform. Even some groups that stand to gain substantially have become preoccupied with specific provisions they don't like and come to think of themselves as victims of change, instead of seizing the opportunities that reform presents. So many complex interests are implicated in health care reform that only strong and articulate national leadership can overcome the powerful emotional as well as economic forces that inhibit us from effective action.

Today, those who play upon fear to preserve the status quo play especially upon distrust of government. One recent study of public opinion about health care quoted a man from Flint, Michigan, who said, "I am for national health care, but I don't want the government involved." Opponents of national health insurance have seized upon the statement as evidence that the public is confused rather than strongly in support of national health insurance. I take the man's position to be entirely reasonable. National health care—yes, in the sense that all citizens must have access to coverage and care. The national government managing health care—no. Even Canada's federal government does not manage the system; in fact, the total number of federal employees concerned with national health insurance in Ottawa is fewer than two dozen.

The alliance model calls for universal health coverage with federal standards, but the organization would be doubly decentralized to the states and the private sector. The states would establish regional authorities to structure the competition; private health plans would deliver services and assume financial risks. The federal law would give the states the flexibility to carry out universal coverage and cost containment through diverse means. A state could decide that a competitive structure does not fit its circumstances and adopt a single-payer system. Providing for diverse solutions not only makes political sense; it is potentially an important source of learning. We will be better off if the states undertake different strategies of reform, even if some fail, than if the nation as a whole continues to be deadlocked because we cannot agree on one system for all.

I said earlier that national health reform is not like a riddle without an answer. Nor is it like a problem in arithmetic, to which there is only one right answer. Around the world are diverse systems of health care finance that appear to perform better than ours, and at home we have many positive examples of alternative ways of organizing insurance and medical care. Public

opinion polls often find majorities for conflicting remedies to the health care crisis, and some observers suggest, therefore, that the polls mean nothing. A more
reasonable interpretation, it seems to me, is that, while
not understanding the technicalities, many Americans
feel they could probably live with more than one approach. But they want their leaders to act.

Many people today are skeptical that the federal government can act rationally on health insurance or, for
that matter, on anything else. Opponents of reform call
upon that cynicism to discourage strong, comprehensive
action. In a sense, they have laid down a challenge to democratic government: Are we simply destined to let the
crisis of health costs and health insurance unfold? Or
can we finally arrive at positive agreement on reform after decades of stalemate? When he introduced his plan
for reform, President Clinton did not merely summon
Americans to undertake a great "national journey." He
set out a clear vision of where the journey should take
us and how we are most likely to get there. Now we
must begin.

FOR THE BEST IN PAPERBACKS, LOOK FOR THE 🐧

In every corner of the world, on every subject under the sun, Penguin represents quality and variety—the very best in publishing today.

For complete information about books available from Penguin—including Pelicans, Puffins, Peregrines, and Penguin Classics—and how to order them, write to us at the appropriate address below. Please note that for copyright reasons the selection of books varies from country to country.

In the United Kingdom: For a complete list of books available from Penguin in the U.K., please write to *Dept E.P., Penguin Books Ltd, Harmondsworth, Middlesex, UB7 0DA.*

In the United States: For a complete list of books available from Penguin in the U.S., please write to *Consumer Sales, Penguin USA, P.O. Box 999—Dept. 17109, Bergenfield, New Jersey 07621-0120.* VISA and MasterCard holders call 1-800-253-6476 to order all Penguin titles.

In Canada: For a complete list of books available from Penguin in Canada, please write to *Penguin Books Canada Ltd, 10 Alcorn Avenue, Suite 300, Toronto, Ontario, Canada M4V 3B2.*

In Australia: For a complete list of books available from Penguin in Australia, please write to the *Marketing Department, Penguin Books Ltd, P.O. Box 257, Ringwood, Victoria 3134.*

In New Zealand: For a complete list of books available from Penguin in New Zealand, please write to the *Marketing Department, Penguin Books (NZ) Ltd, Private Bag, Takapuna, Auckland 9.*

In India: For a complete list of books available from Penguin, please write to *Penguin Overseas Ltd, 706 Eros Apartments, 56 Nehru Place, New Delhi, 110019.*

In Holland: For a complete list of books available from Penguin in Holland, please write to *Penguin Books Nederland B.V., Postbus 195, NL-1380AD Weesp, Netherlands.*

In Germany: For a complete list of books available from Penguin, please write to *Penguin Books Ltd, Friedrichstrasse 10-12, D-6000 Frankfurt Main I, Federal Republic of Germany.*

In Spain: For a complete list of books available from Penguin in Spain, please write to *Longman, Penguin España, Calle San Nicolas 15, E-28013 Madrid, Spain.*

In Japan: For a complete list of books available from Penguin in Japan, please write to *Longman Penguin Japan Co Ltd, Yamaguchi Building, 2-12-9 Kanda Jimbocho, Chiyoda-Ku, Tokyo 101, Japan.*